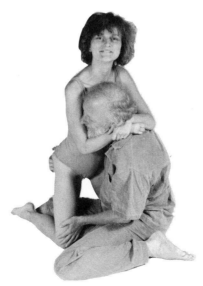

This book is dedicated to Valerie

Published by
Harbin Springs Publishing,. P. O. Box 82, Middletown, CA 95461

First Printing: October, 1987
Second Printing: February, 1991

1. Acupressure. 2. Massage. I. Title.
RM723.A27D85 1987 613.7 87-82475
ISBN 0-944202-00-4

Printed in the United States of America

BODYWORK

TANTRA

ON

LAND

AND

IN

WATER

CO-CENTERING

WATSU

TANTSU

BY

HAROLD

DULL

with move montages by the author

ACKNOWLEDGMENTS

I would like to acknowledge and express my gratitude to those whose assistance have made this work and this book possible: to the woman who gave me my first massage beside a hot spring one day; to my three teachers- Reuho Yamada, Wataru Ohashi and Shizuto Masunaga; to my wife, Valerie, whose love has been a constant support and who is the model for the Tantsu and Watsu pictures in this book; to my students who have put so much into the creating of these patterns; to my assistant, Elaine Marie, who has put her heart into getting Watsu out to as many people as possible; to Ann Prehn who took the photos in this book; to Libby Hillman who set the type; to Ishvara and all the rest at Harbin who have made this the kind of place where this could be developed.

The School and the Place

Harbin Hot Springs, an ancient Native American healing site, and a once-famous, turn-of-the-century resort, is now home to a community of a hundred and fifty who maintain it as a New Age retreat and workshop center. It is also home to the School of Shiatsu and Massage where students come from all over the world for workshops and intensive training and certification programs in Bodywork Tantra.

Surrounded by 1160 acres of its own mountains, valley, streams and woods, and with its own natural hot springs and pools, Harbin Hot Springs is a place of rare peace and beauty, an ideal setting for the kinds of growth and transformation the school's programs facilitate. Set up as a church of 'Being' with the doctrine that everyone is free to pursue their own spiritual path, Harbin is officially known as 'Heart Consciousness Church'. It is not surprising that this is the place where a bodywork that emphasizes 'being with someone' and 'heart consciousness' and freedom would be developed.

For information about the school and its programs, about videos and tapes to accompany this book, or about our workshop programs around the world, please write THE SCHOOL OF SHIATSU AND MASSAGE, Box 570, Middletown, CA 95461.

PREFACE

This is a do-it-yourselves bodywork book.

You are about to learn step by step patterns that have been tested and evolved in hundreds of classes. Practicing these simple patterns over and over you will begin to feel a greater connection to others and become more aware of the different forms and states of energy in your own body. You will come to feel how bodywork can be a practice for your own development much in the way that meditation, tai chi and yoga are practices; but a practice in which you connect to and help others get in touch with their own centers and energies.

The bodywork in this book differs from traditional shiatsu in that equal importance is placed on working with meridians and chakras. The system of meridians (and the acupuncture points they connect) reached its fullest development in China; the system of chakras (our major energy centers), in Tibet and India. The more elaborate the theories built up around these two systems the less compatible they are. But that both chakras and meridians have a real existence in our bodies, and that there is an intimate connection between them, becomes more apparent the more you practice Bodywork Tantra.

Rather than presenting the theories behind either system in their elaborated forms (there are many other books in which you can find these), this book presents the common denominator of the two, that which has been most supported by what I, and those I have worked with, have felt in our own bodies. This is a feel-it-yourselves book and the more you practice Bodywork Tantra the more you will understand in your own body just what meridians and chakras are. It is impossible to work on someone else's chakras without engaging, and consequently working on your own. This is the basis of our practice.

An 'Anatomy of Energy', which follows this book's patterns, integrates discussions of each chakra and its related meridians with meditations to further help you get in touch with them. Practice these meditations as you learn the patterns in this book. It is followed by an 'Autobiography of Energy' which relates other experiences and practices of Tantra.

CONTENTS

Preface

INTRODUCTION

Tantra 9
Zen Shiatsu 9
Watsu   10
Tantsu   10
Co-centering 10

PREPARATIONS

The mother hand 11
Center holding 11
Preparing body, heart and mind 12
Preparing the place and the person 13
Caution 13

CO-CENTERING

Basic Co-Centering 15
Expanded Co-centering 21
The Hara 28

WATSU

Introduction 31
Preparations 32
Nine Watsu Lessons
I The Basic Rock 34
II The Leg Rotations 36
III The Far Leg Over 38
IV The Near Leg Over 40
V Basic Finishes 42
VI The Stepwork 44
VII The Gyroscope 46
VIII The Wallwork 48
IX Freestyle 50

BASIC TANTSU

Tantsu 53
The Side 54
The Leg Cradle 58
The Turtle 60
The Lap 62

FURTHER EXPANSIONS OF CO-CENTERING

Face Down from above the Head 64
The Co-Centering Side 66
The Sitting 68

EXPANDING THE TANTSU

The Expanded Tantsu Side 70
The Expanded Lap 72

FREESTYLE AND FREE FORM 74

THE MERIDIAN STRETCHES 76

AN ANATOMY OF ENERGY

Meditations, CHAKRAS, Meridian Pairs
The Void, THE TAO, Bladder/Kidney 78
The One, THE CROWN, The Central Meridians 80
The Inside, THE HEART CHAKRA, Heart/Small Intestine 82
The Two, The Meridian Pairs, Circulation/Triple Heater 84
The Three, THE NAVEL CHAKRA, Stomach/Spleen 86
The Ten Thousand, THE POWER CHAKRA, Gall Bladder/Liver 88
The Balance, THE THROAT CHAKRA, THE THIRD EYE 90
Lung/Large Intestine 91
The Meridian Pairs and their Associations 92

A NOTE ON DIAGNOSIS 94

AN AUTOBIOGRAPHY OF ENERGY 96

CIRCLES CELEBRATING CONNECTION 105

The Tao gives birth to the one...
The One gives birth to the Two...
The Two gives birth to the Three...
And the Three to the Ten Thousand...

Lao Tzu

INTRODUCTION

The Master of Tantra, poet William Blake, writes 'Energy is eternal delight.' It is when it's flowing freely through our body. When it's rushing up our back and settling back into our center, when it's swirling around our heart and shining clearly in our mind, it is ecstasy. And when we feel its connection to the universe, it is enlightenment.

But when it's blocked, when it's locked in tension, when our hearts close and our minds narrow, it is pain. And we feel alone and cut off from others.

Tantra is the practice of freeing this energy, through centering, opening chakras and unblocking its flow. This can be done individually (meditation and yoga), with intimate partners (Tantra of Union), or with anybody (Bodywork Tantra).

Zen Shiatsu

My introduction to this kind of bodywork was Zen Shiatsu, which I first studied with the Zen priest Reuho Yamada. He once referred to it as Zen Tantra. It had been developed by the author of 'Zen Shiatsu,' Shizuto Masunaga, who I was later to study with in Japan. It combines traditional Japanese shiatsu (pressing the same points used in acupuncture) with stretching and other oriental techniques to release and balance the energy in the meridians (the pathways connecting the points).

Masunaga speaks of establishing a 'life echo' with whoever we work with. Practicing this I began to feel a connection with others that had been missing in my life. And I became more centered and aware of the energy coursing through my own meridians. He also speaks of the person we are working with as being our 'teacher' in our paths to enlightenment. He emphasizes 'being with' rather than 'doing something to' that person, of remaining 'empty' and following their need.

Built into this eclectic bodywork is a spirit of freedom and creativity, which can lead to a multitude of styles. Reuho Yamada developed his own called 'New Age Shiatsu' and another teacher I studied with, Wataru Ohashi, developed what he called 'Ohashiatsu.'

Watsu

When I began to teach Zen Shiatsu, I tried to teach separately the various styles and forms of my three teachers, but found it confused my students. In my own practice I had already combined them in a way natural to me and I began to teach this. At the same time I began to apply some of the stretches and moves of Zen Shiatsu while floating people in the warm pool at Harbin Hot Springs.

As people relax into the warm water, they are more open to stretching. They feel the total support water provides. Constant flowing movement releases tension from the spine. There is an incredible sense of being nurtured and a womb-like peace. Many people speak of moving into altered states of consciousness. When the chakras are held, both parties become more aware of the energy in them and often feel a movement up the spine.

In Wat(er Shiat)su I found that, holding someone in water, I felt an even stronger connection to them than on land.

Bodywork is a celebration of connection!

Tantsu

I wanted to duplicate on land Watsu's connection and nurturing and power, and developed a form in which we use our whole body to hold and cradle someone from beginning to end. The more you are held the more you can let go. It is done in dance-like patterns, each move flowing into the next, in a way that further encourages someone to completely let go. Because, besides releasing points and stretching meridians, it focuses on connecting chakras and freeing the energy moving up the spine, it is called Tant(ric Shiat)su.

Co-centering

To make things easier for my students, I needed a form that, practicing, would teach them to lean in and to hold with their whole body; a form they could learn in a few hours but one complete enough to give that feeling at the end, when the hands are lifted off, of there still being a connection.

I found that a form based on continuously working out from and returning to the body's three basic centers (the centers of body, heart and mind) was simple enough to learn and teach others, but still so effective and powerful you become more centered the more you practice it. Because it centers the giver as well as the receiver it is called Co-centering.

With the help of students in hundreds of classes we evolved and fine tuned the Basic Co-centering form that appears in this book. It is an ideal introduction to shiatsu. In addition it is a framework within which to incorporate the more detailed point-work and stretches of the expanded forms which follow it.

Centering the body, opening the heart, clearing the mind...the more you work on others the more you work on yourself. When you hold someone and feel their surrender and your connection to them it is hard to maintain a judgemental or superior attitude. When you feel them letting go of tension and the fear behind it, it is hard to hold onto your own fears. And when you feel how the tension that is released with one hand is energy that goes through your center and out your other hand to wherever it is needed without 'draining' you, you will find it easier to just be with someone and stay empty without trying to do anything to them. And at the end of a session you will feel a peace, a calm in which you have more centered, loving and clear energy than before. Bodywork Tantra is a practice. Whoever we work with is our teacher...the one who can help us to higher states of awareness and realization of our own being.

The Mother Hand

If you reach out and poke one point after another, a person feels alternately invaded and abandoned. He feels pain. If one hand leans into a point with a gentle constant presence while the other hand, in coordination with the breathing, leans into one point after another, a person feels supported throughout. He feels his body is being worked on as a whole and is able to accept deeper and more effective penetration without pain or resistance.

The hand that remains constant in one place is called 'the mother hand'. It facilitates your connecting, leaning in and working with your whole body. You can prepare yourself to use the mother hand. First do the meridian-pair stretches described on page 76. Then sit and do the meditation described on page 78, letting everything settle into your center as you breathe out...

Keeping the sense of everything emptying into your center everytime you breathe out, get up on all fours, your knees about a foot apart. With your arms straight, rock forward as you breathe out, and back as you breathe in(Rock just far enough back to where it requires no effort to rock forward again). Everytime you rock forward feel the letting go in your neck and spine and the settling into your center. Still rocking, place your right hand alongside your left. As you rock forward lean your increasing weight into your right hand. As you rock back keep the weight in your left hand constant as your right hand moves away a couple of inches. Keep your left constant as you rock forward into your right again. The weight leaning into your left hand is a constant, midway between the zero and the full weight leaning into your other hand. After leaning into three different places with your right start it again alongside your mother hand. Continue. Feel how your left hand becomes attached to the floor and how the weight in the right gradually increases the full length of the outbreath as you let go more and more into your center.

Center Holding

When you use the mother hand this way and connect to someone's breathing, you feel the letting go in your own center as you lean in with each outbreath. Leaning in some places, you feel a less complete letting go. Those are where you need to stay longer than one breath. And as you stay, the person feels your presence as truly 'being' with him, and can open up and release more. Connected to someone this way you begin to intuitively go places that need holding...and stay as long as needed. This is the basis of a 'good touch.' We find the 'points' with our center, not with our fingertips or a chart.

A simple experiment can demonstrate the power of center holding. Have someone sit looking away, his arm on the floor. Hold his forearm with both hands, your fingers under, and your thumbs on top side by side. Press. It will feel to him like one point. A set distance is required between two points for them to no longer feel like one. To find that distance separate your thumbs slightly and press as if looking for something (Press with your brain). Keep separating your thumbs and pressing until he feels two points. When the set distance (which in laboratory experiments has proven to be a constant) is determined, start again. This time prepare yourself with a centering meditation. Let everything empty into the bottom of your hara. The more centered you become, the farther apart you will be able to move your thumbs before he feels them holding separate places, the more he will feel the unity and connection in his body...and the more you will feel it in your own body.

Preparing Body

Practicing Bodywork Tantra you will experience your own body becoming more centered and vibrant and supple. Do not try to force this process. If you feel any discomfort in any of the positions in this book, accustom yourself to them gradually.

If you are not used to seiza (sitting on your heels) you can use rolled up towels (under your ankles) or cushions to help get used to this position. Sitting on a meditation bench at a low table while reading or writing is a way to get your knees used to being bent for periods of time. Hatha Yoga helps prepare your body for all these positions.

Don't push your body into any position it is not comfortable in. If you are uncomfortable and unable to completely let go yourself, the person you work with will not be able to either. If you are unable to work on the floor much of this can be adapted to a massage table.

In whatever position you're in take advantage of your own body's weight and leverage. Use as little muscle power as possible. When possible use your muscles in a state of tonus, the effortless state they're in when you walk down the street carrying a briefcase. While working, regularly check your own position and posture. The more you practice this bodywork, the more your own posture will improve.

Preparing Heart

The more you practice Bodywork Tantra the more you will experience an opening of the heart center. The more accepting of others you will become; the more you will feel your connection to every other person.

Accept others where they are at. Do not try to force bodywork on anybody. Accept that there are many people who are not ready to let go of tension. Accept that they have a reason to carry it, that we all create our own reality. And that each person's reality is his own creation and has its own inner logic and is beautiful.

Welcome however much or however little each person is ready to let go in your arms. Accept it as a gift. Cherish the trust they place in you. Celebrate connection.

Preparing Mind

The more practiced you become, the more ingrained the bodywork sequences become, the more intuitive (with 'no mind') you hold and move from place to place, the greater clarity you will experience in your mind center.

In Bodywork Tantra we support someone with the centered strength of our hara. We support them with the loving acceptance of our heart. And we support them with the clarity expressed in the effortless flowing dancelike continuity of our moves from beginning to end.

At first the process of learning can get in the way of developing this clarity. Go slowly. This book is set up so that you can proceed bit by bit. Learn each step thoroughly before you go on to the next. And you will find an increasing clarity as you practice over and over the sequences in this book.

And at the end of a session as you hold and connect someone's heart center and third eye and feel the energy straightening and rising up your own back, feel how much greater clarity there is in your own mind center.

Preparing Place

A large floor with a well padded rug is ideal. The room should be well heated and free of drafts. Lay out a sheet to work on. Have a rolled up towel nearby. And a blanket to cover the person afterwards.

On warm days you can work outside as long as you take precautions not to have too much sun on your own head. Both you and the person you work with should be wearing loose clothes which do not interfere with the stretches.

Preparing the person

Find out what his previous experiences with bodywork have been and what kind of pressure he likes. Ask him if he has any questions about shiatsu. Give him the feeling that you know what you are doing and put him as much at his ease as possible. Just before starting tell him to let you know if anything is uncomfortable. Tell him that it should feel good. If he has had no experience with bodywork, tell him that it is common for many different kinds of feelings to come up during a session, anger, sadness, desire, etc., and that the thing to do is just to be aware of them, accept them, and let them pass.

Caution

Do not work on someone who has any serious conditions which could be worsened by either pressure or stretching. Do not work on someone who has been bedridden (there is a danger of thrombosis) or whose bones are brittle, from calcium loss. If the person is reccuperating from an illness, work very gently.

Before starting sit and talk with the person. Find out if he has any injuries or health problems which might be aggravated or made worse by pressure or stretching. Ask him if he has any problems with his back or neck or any place else that would limit your pressure or stretching. If he does, avoid those areas. Find out if he would be comfortable in the positions you plan to use. Substitute other positions for those he would be uncomfortable in.

BASIC CO-CENTERING

Basic Co-Centering is a simple but complete form that you can learn in a few hours and begin practicing on others. No previous knowledge of bodywork, points or meridians is needed. The more you practice this the more you will feel the connection in your own center(s). The more you feel this connection the more you will know intuitively where to go and how long to stay.

Practice this over and over until you feel it completely ingrained in your body before you go on to learn the Expanded Co-centering or the Tantsu. Be attentive to how you are using your body. Are you in the most comfortable position possible? Is it a position which allows you to let go, to settle into your own center as you lean in? The more you can let go the more the person you are working with can let go. Feel the letting go in your hara center.

Co-Centering is centering with a person. It is also the connecting of each person's centers: body to heart to mind. When you sit alongside someone, one hand reaching across your hara to hold his hara and the other hand coming from your heart to his heart, both you, and your Co-centering partner, are experiencing a greater connection between these centers. And the connection between that center and the meridians related to it is strengthened when you keep one hand on the center while the other works out arm or leg.

After working out from one center and returning to its connection to another center, you will often feel the center you have just worked out from more open and at higher level of energy then the one you haven't yet worked out from. Do not try to move energy from the higher to the lower. Just sit and hold both, keeping empty yourself, and you will feel the lower gradually approach the level of the higher. And each time you return to their connection, you will feel both becoming stronger and more open.

And when heart and mind are connected at the end you will often feel the movement up the spine that connects all three, and connects us each to a higher reality.

Make sure he has no problems pressure or stretching could aggravate. Have him lie face down, his arms comfortably out to the sides, his head turned. Place a rolled up towel under his upper chest to see if it makes him more comfortable. (If he is not comfortable lying face down do not work on him in this position but start instead with him lying on his back, number 9 in these notes. Later you will learn other ways to work on the back.) Tell him to feel free to turn his head whenever he wants and to let you know if anything is uncomfortable. Sit seiza (on your heels) facing his lower back, your knees a couple inches from his left side. Center yourself.

1. **The Opening Rock.** Simultaneously place your left hand across his spine between the shoulder blades (behind the heart chakra) and your right hand across his lower back just above the sacrum. Without leaning in, hold for three breaths, connecting to his breathing. On an inbreath place your left hand alongside your right hand. As he breathes out lean into the muscle a couple inches to this side of the spine with the heels of both hands (the angle of your lean more towards the spine than towards the floor). With the next outbreath hook your fingers into the corresponding muscle on the other side of his spine and rock back. Still sitting on your heels, keep your arms and back straight, and rock from your center. With your hands maintaining a bowed curve rock their heels into the muscle and rock back with hooked fingers gradually building up to that individuals most natural rate of rocking. Maintaining the rock with both hands let your left hand walk up by letting your heel lift up when the fingers hook in and your fingers lift up when your heel leans in, letting them move up the spine a fraction of an inch with each rock. When it is a few inches up from the right hand jump it back and start it walking up again without breaking rhythm. This time let it walk a little higher before jumping it back and starting over. The third time let it walk up to where you placed it at the very beginning. Gradually slow the rocking down to a stop. Feel the slowing down in your own hara. Hold three breaths.

2. **The Lean Down the Near Side.** Keeping your left hand over his heart center, get up on both knees spreading and moving them far enough back from him to be able to rock forward comfortably with your weight. Place the heel of your right hand just below your left hand to the near side of his spine. Breathe out as he breathes out and lean into your right hand. Rock back as you both breathe in, sliding your hand down three or four inches. Lean in again on the next outbreath. Do this again in one more place; this last should be in the lower back just above the sacrum. Keep leaning into your left hand (the mother hand) throughout with a constant pressure midway between the zero and the full weight of your right hand. The pressure of your right hand should be vertical and applied about an inch to an inch and a half to this side of the spine. It should be painless. There should be no pressure on the spine. Keep both arms straight and relaxed. Feel the letting go at the bottom of each breath in your own center. Start again at the top and repeat, leaning into the three places. Repeat a third time.

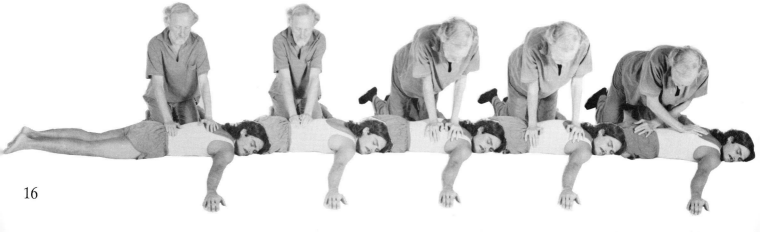

3. **The Lean Down the Far Side.** Slip the heel of your left hand to the other side of his spine and, placing the heel of your right hand below it, repeat the above to the far side of the spine, three places three times. Rock far enough across to maintain vertical pressure (You may need to move in a little closer).

4. **The Crossed Arm Stretch.** Move your right hand from its last position just above the sacrum onto the middle of the spine as you cross your left hand under your right arm onto the sacrum. Lean gradually into both, pushing apart, stretching the spine. Hold through one outbreath.

5. **The Lean down Buttock and Thigh.** Lean constantly into the sacrum with the heel of your left hand as the heel of your right hand leans vertically into the middle of the left buttock, into the top of the leg (the base of the thumb pressing up under the buttock), and into the very middle of the thigh. Repeat leaning into these three places two more times.

6. **The Foot Press.** Swing up his left foot. Keep leaning your weight into his sacrum with your left hand while your right hand, holding his foot just above the toes, gently presses his left heel towards his left buttock.

7. **The Far Leg.** Lay his leg out straight and, keeping your left hand on his sacrum, repeat the above three places, three times, down the right buttock and leg (You are still on his left side).

8. **The Roll Over.** After pressing his right leg towards his buttock, hold his foot just above the right side of his ankle. With your left hand carefully slide his left arm up alongside his head. Reach across and slide his right arm (palm up) down to his side. Holding his wrist from underneath, pull his right arm up and back, rolling him onto his back (your right hand pulling, straightening and lowering his right leg).

9. **The Hara Rock.** Sit seiza alongside his hara (to his right). Make sure his legs, arms and neck are straight and his head is in line with the body. Cross your left hand onto his hara (from your hara) just below the navel, and your right hand onto his heart chakra (from your heart). Connect to his breathing. Hold at least three breaths. Lay both hands flat on the hara (they shouldn't be crossing the midline and they shouldn't be so close to either the ribs or the pelvis that they pull skin when you lean in). Gently and slowly rocking in from your own hara with each outbreath, cup your hands down and in towards the center. Watch his face for any signs of discomfort. Continue for several breaths. Place your left hand back across the hara (below the navel), and your right hand on the heart chakra. Hold.

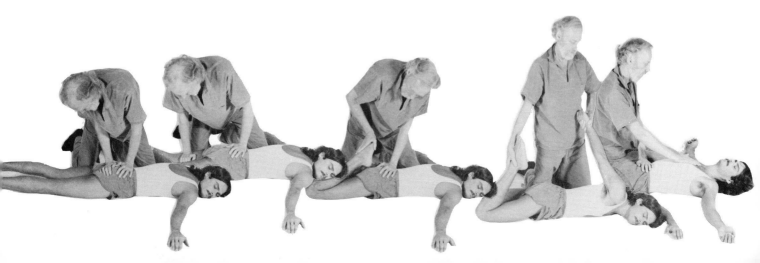

10. **The Lean out the Arm.** Get up on your knees, keeping your right hand on his heart center, without leaning any body weight into it. As he breathes out gently lean the heel of your left hand into his chest just below the shoulder. On the next outbreath lean into the lower arm where it is widest (a third of the way down from the elbow and a little to the outside). On the next outbreath lean into the middle of his palm. Have yourself positioned far enough back, your knees spread and your arms straight, so that you can gradually lean in with your weight instead of using your 'muscles'. Watch his face for any reaction. Lean into these three places two more times. Keeping your right hand on his heart center and your left on his palm, sit back alongside his hara. Cross your left hand back onto his hara. Hold for at least three breaths feeling the energy between these two centers balance (the energy in whichever is lower rise to the level of the higher).

11. **The Lean down the Leg.** Get up on your knees, keeping your left hand on his hara (just below the navel). On the outbreath lean the heel of your right hand into the top of his leg (a little to the outside). On the next outbreath lean into his leg just above his knee (to the outside where it mounds up). Leaning in from the side, lean into the leg just below the knee. Repeat two more times.

12. **The Leg Roll.** Keeping your left hand on his hara, place your right hand on the outside of his right thigh and gently roll his leg at a speed at which the momentum of his foot adds to the roll. Continue the rolling as your hand works down to his foot.

13. **The Foot Rotation.** Pick up his right foot and move into a position sitting seiza under it so that the curve just above his heel fits smoothly across your upper left thigh (you are facing his other foot). Hold it close to your hara with your left hand holding the ankle (from above) and your right hand holding his foot (from below). Your left thumb and forefinger should have a pincer hold in the depressions just below the malleolus. Rotate and stretch his foot, circling with your body. Change directions as you wish.

14. **The Leg Rotation.** With your left hand tuck up his pants if necessary and lift up under his knee moving back to his right side, your left knee raised, your right knee on the floor. Holding the top of his knee with your left hand and the bottom of his foot with your right, press his knee towards his right shoulder. Gently rotate in a circle outward from his chest.

15. **The Leg Rock.** Gradually straightening his leg, stand and, facing him, hold his foot to the inside of your right leg, your left hand holding his heel and your right hand the top of his foot. Leaning back, rock in a direction away from him.

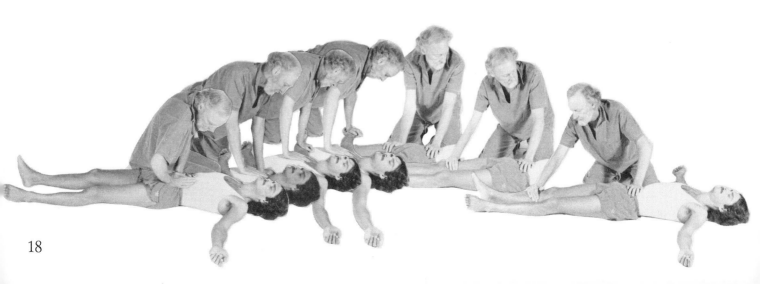

16. **The Knees Press.** With your left hand bend his right knee as your right hand picks up his left leg (from below the knee, tucking up his pants leg if necessary). Straddling his legs, press both knees towards his chest keeping his sacrum flat on the floor (your hands pressing his legs just below the knees). Hold at least three breaths. Lower his legs and, sitting alongside his left side, place your right hand on his hara and your left on his heart center. Hold. Work out his left arm, return to the hara and work down his left leg (a mirror image of the above).

17. **The Swing.** (Optional) After finishing the second Leg Rock, hold both his knees pressed back up towards his chest (as in 16). Bend your knees. Straighten his legs and hold his heels (or calves) to the front of your chest. Straighten your legs, lifting him up by the legs (still clasped to your chest) without straining your back. If his sacrum easily lifts off the floor, slowly swing him from side to side. Continue swinging him as you gradually lower his spine to the floor.

18. **The Leg Pull.** Holding his legs by the heels (keeping them straight), squat back and pull both legs. Lower his feet to the floor and lean into the tops (just below the toes), stretching his feet down.

19. **The Crossed Arm Pull.** Walk up along his left side, picking up his left wrist with your right hand. Moving above his head, pick up his right wrist with your left hand. Cross his arms and squat back to pull. Lay both arms back out to his sides.

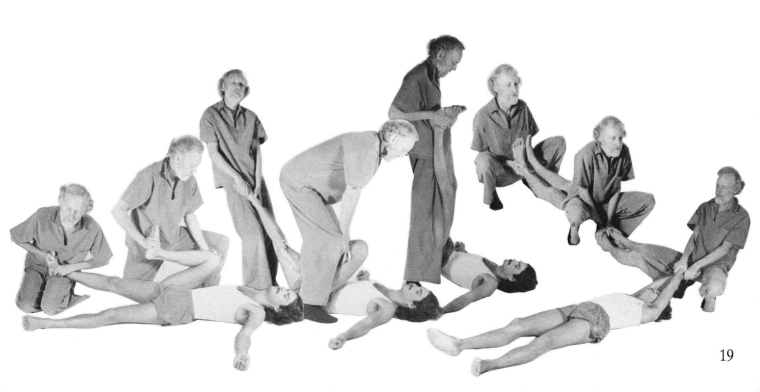

19

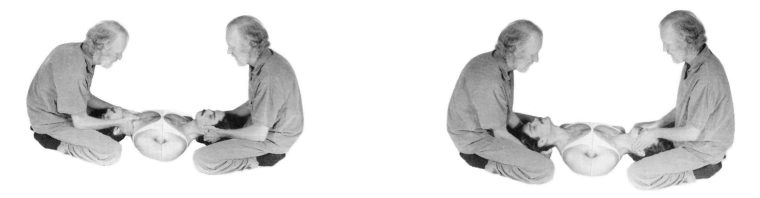

20. **The Neck Wave.** Sit seiza above his head. Starting with your fingertips under the base of his neck, lift up with a gentle rolling wave without sliding on the skin. Repeat two more places working up to just under the occiput. Repeat three times.

21. **The Head Pull.** Hold his head in your hands, the sides of your fingers under his occiput. Keeping his neck straight, lean back to pull.

22. **The Occiput Hold.** Hold under the occiput with all eight fingers letting his chin raise and his head fall back not quite touching the floor. (The backs of your hands are resting on the floor.) Hold. Lower.

23. **The Eye Cupping.** Place your cupped hands (fingers outward) across his face, blocking out all light to his eyes (without touching them).

24. **The Finish.** Simultaneously lay your left hand across his forehead(over his third eye) and your right hand(fingers pointing towards his feet) over his heart chakra. Hold at least three breaths feeling the energy balance between these two centers. At the same time be aware of your own back, its straightness and the energy moving up it. Slowly lift off both hands and 'sit' feeling how you are still connected...and how you are seperate.

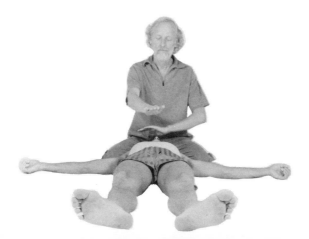

EXPANDED CO-CENTERING

In the following expansion you begin to incorporate more detailed pointwork within the framework of the basic pattern. You will continue to utilize the Basic Move (the leaning into three places with the heel of your hand) to open up and get a feel for the pathways (and to establish your mother hand). Instead of repeating it three times, do it once and then work down the same meridian (which your mother hand continues holding) with elbow or thumb.

Using the elbow, which does not work as intimately with the brain as the thumb does, encourages you to get out of your head and work from your body center. Place your right elbow in the center of your left hand. Move it around. Feel how the looser skin it is sheathed in gives it more freedom of movement than your thumb has when it is placed there. Place your elbow on the back of your fingers. Feel how it slips right in between two fingers. When working down the back if it lands on a bone it will slip between it and the next, which is where the points are.

Place your elbow back in your hand and feel the difference when your right arm is more, or less, bent. The more bent the arm, the sharper the elbow. In the following keep your arm less bent and your wrist limp. You want your arm as free of tension as possible.

When working with your thumb, lean in with the flatter part just under the tip rather than the sharper tip. When working out an arm or leg, use the rest of your hand to hold the arm or leg when possible. To arrive at the point, slide your thumb up until you feel its indentation or, with practice, a sense of arrival at a point. This sense is greatly facilitated by the use of the mother hand and connected breathing. Holding a point, feel its release in your own hara. If you do not feel the completion at the bottom of your breath, stay with it longer, riding over the breath, i.e. keep a steady pressure as he breathes in and sink in a little deeper as he breathes out. Normally we work with a steady pressure (within the person's limits). Occasionally you will feel points that need some movement or vibration to help release them.

The points are referred to by number and their locations can be found on the meridian charts and their accompanying descriptions later in this book.

In the following sequence you will be working the meridians in their traditional direction - the yin upward and the yang downward (the arms raised).

As in all the work in this book, encourage the recipient to provide feedback and keep you informed of any discomfort.

The Expanded Face Down

Sit facing his back and rock as in Basic. Hold.

1. **Both Hands down the Back.** Sit facing his back and rock as in Basic. Hold. Get up on your knees and place both hands (fingers pointed outwards) between his spine and shoulder blades. Tell him to take a deep breath and let it all the way out. As he breathes out lean into the heels of both hands. As he breathes in slide both hands a few inches down and lean in again. Repeat in a third place. Don't go past the rib cage into the lower back. As he breathes in place both hands, one above the other to the far side of the spine and, keeping the left hand mothering, lean into three places as in Basic.

2. **Elbow Far Side.** Keeping the heel of your left hand on the bladder meridian between his right scapula and spine, work with your right elbow (arm open) down the bladder meridian (1-1 & 1/2 inches to the right of his spine) to just above his sacrum, leaning into the points alongside (between) each vertebra.

3. **The Near Side.** Slip your mother hand to the left side of his spine and lean into three places down this side of the spine with the heel of your right hand as in Basic.

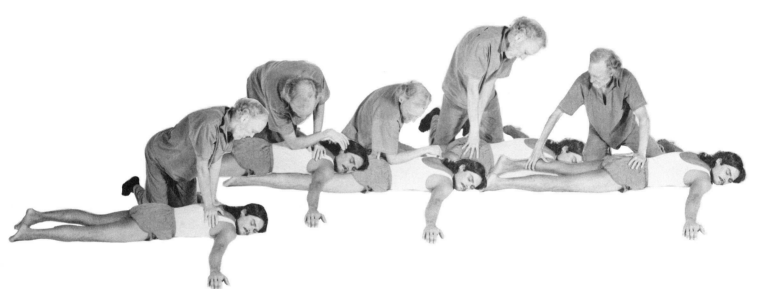

Keep your mother hand in the upper back and, sitting seiza alongside his back, work down the near side of his spine, leaning in with your right elbow.

4. **The Sacrum.** When your elbow is in the last point just above his sacrum, keep it there as you reach behind it with your left thumb onto the first point on the sacrum. Placing your right thumb on the corresponding point on the right side of his sacrum, get up on both knees and (still facing his head), leaning in at an angle perpindicular to the sacrum, lean into the points in the foramen(the small indentations in the back of the sacrum) and to the sides of the tailbone with both thumbs. Place your left hand on his sacrum and your right hand on the spine where it curves up. Lean in to cross stretch as in Basic.

5. **Legs and Calves.** Keeping your mother hand on the sacrum lean in once with the heel of your hand into the buttock, the top of the leg and the middle of the thigh (as in Basic); and once with your elbow... Then with your right thumb slide lightly down the back of the calf (between the muscles), stopping three times to hold a point. Swing up and press his foot towards his buttock, as in Basic. Repeat the above leaning across to the far side and then, taking his ankle, roll him over as in Basic.

6. **Out the Right Arm.** Sitting alongside his right side, place your left hand on his hara and your right hand on his Heart Center. Hold. Work the Hara here as in Basic, rocking in from your own center. (It is here where the expanded work on the hara described in the next section is to be inserted.) Place your right hand back on the heart center. Up on your knees, keeping your right hand on his heart center, lean your left hand into his chest, lower arm and palm as in Basic.

7. **Lung.** Keeping his arm on the floor, slide it down (still straight) to between your knees. Hold Lung 9 (in his wrist below the thumb) with your left thumb while your right thumb works lung points down the arm (Lung 3,5 and 6). While holding these points your fingers should be holding the arm from underneath (His arm stays on the floor during this and the next move).

8. **Large Intestine.** Hold Large Intestine 4 in the side of his hand with your left thumb, your left hand bending his wrist forward, while the four fingers of your right hand clasp Large Intestine 8, 9, 10 and 11 in the side of the forearm (where you feel the stretch). Hold.

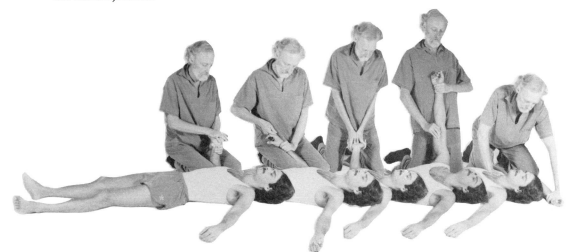

9. **Wrist and Fingers.** With your left hand hold his wrist and swing his lower arm up (your knees are straddling his elbow). Stretch his wrist back and forth. Rotate. Pull his fingers one at a time(his hand lying across your thigh).

10. **The Hand Weave.** Open his hand by slipping your last two fingers of each hand between his fingers (your hands facing his hands, a little finger to each side of his middle finger) and, up on your knees (his elbow between them), lean both thumbs into the middle of his palm (Circulation 8).

11. **Circulation.** Hold his wrist with your left hand and, holding his arm to your chest, rock up and back. With the first rock, the four fingers of your right hand press into the front of the arm just past the shoulder as your thumb squeezes the back of the arm. Between each rock your hand slips a little higher up the midline (Circulation and Triple Heater meridians) until after four or five rocks it has reached the wrist.

12. **Heart.** Lay his arm up above his head (Heart Meridian stretch). Mother Heart 1 in the middle of his armpit with your right hand (flat and without pressure) while your left palm just under your fingers very lightly leans into a couple of places in the upper arm and a couple in the lower. Lower his arm back out to his side.

13. **Leg**. Lean into his hand with your left hand while your right hand returns to his heart center. Sitting seiza alongside him, place your left hand on his hara. Hold. Up on your knees, keeping your left hand on his hara, work down and roll his leg as in Basic.

14. **Stomach**. End the leg roll pressing his right foot down and inward. Hold it turned that way with your right knee (without excess pressure) as you place your left thumb in Stomach 36. Mother there while your right thumb slides down the Stomach meridian stopping to hold each of the next three points.

15. **Toe Pull**. Lift his right foot and, sitting seiza, hold it in your lap against your hara. Rotate and stretch as in Basic. Come out of the last rotation pulling the big toe. Rock away from his body to pull each toe.

16. **The Circle Hook**. With your right hand push the bottom of his foot (just below the toes) rocking towards his body while the four fingers of your left

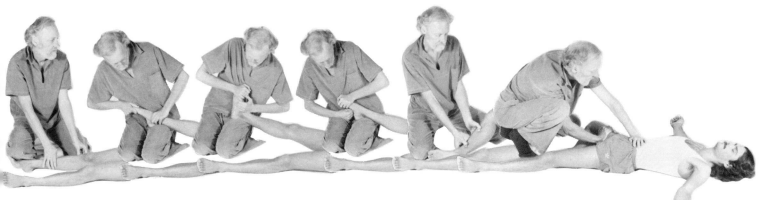

hand hook into the bottom of his foot (in the softer part) and pull with each rock. Between each rock place the fingers so that after four or five rocks they have completed a clockwise circle.

17. **The Rock into the Thumb.** Place your right thumb in the midline of the sole near his heel and, with your left hand holding the top of his foot near the toes, rock his foot onto your thumb. Between each rock place your thumb closer to the toes. Work up to Kidney 1 and hold.

18. **Spleen**. Place his right leg in Spleen stretch (the right foot midway up his calf) and support his right knee with your left knee (You are still sitting seiza). Mother Spleen 6 with your right thumb while your left thumb works Spleen 7,8 and 9 up his lower right leg(along the bone). Lean with the heel of your left hand into the Spleen points just above the knee, in the middle of the thigh, and at the top of the leg. Lay your left hand across the hara (just below the navel), your right thumb still holding Spleen 6.

19. **Liver.** Leave your left hand on his hara to mother. With your right hand slide his foot up between his legs (his knee still bent out but no longer resting on your knee). Raise your right knee and place the heel of your right hand on the liver meridian in his thigh. Beginning just above the knee, lean into three places working up along the underside of the sartorius muscle. Keep the angle of the push parallel to the floor and brace your upper arm with the inside of your right thigh swinging in with your body.

20. **Kidney.** Keeping your left hand on his hara, swing his still bent knee up with your right hand. Keep your left knee on the floor and position your right knee leaning into his thigh just below the buttock and slightly to the outside (the Kidney meridian on Masunaga's chart). Keeping your knee leaning in, wrap your right arm around his still bent right knee and pull it towards you.

21. **The Leg Press.** From the outside slide your right hand (facing his

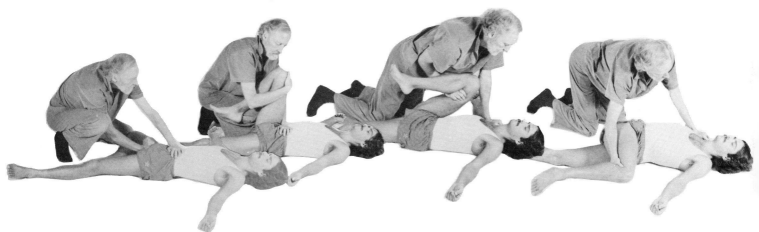

thigh) between his thigh and his calf. Move your left hand from his hara onto his right shoulder and, with both your knees on the floor, push his right knee towards his right shoulder.

22. **The Twist.** Keeping his shoulder held down gently push his bent right knee across his left leg (towards the opposite wall) twist stretching his back.

23. **Basic Leg Work.** Raise your left knee and, holding the bottom of his foot in your right hand and his knee in your left, rotate his leg up towards the chest and away. Standing, hold his foot to the inside of your right thigh and rock away from him as in Basic. Keeping his sacrum flat on the floor, press both his knees towards his chest. Move to his left side. Work a mirror image of the above on arm and leg. After pressing his knees back to his chest, do the Swing, the Leg Pull, the Crossed Arm Pull, the Neck Wave, the Head Pull and the Occiput Hold of Basic.

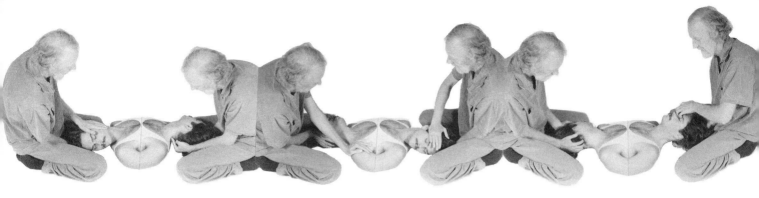

24. **The Neck Work.** Turn his head to both sides (laterally). Turn it back to whatever side it turns easiest towards. Hold the underside of the head with one hand (your fingers hooked into the occiput) while the extended fingers of the other hand work down the neck alongside the vertebra. Your hand under the head moves the head gently bending the neck over the fingers of the other hand. Turn the head and work the other side.

25. **The Neck Stretches.** Push his head (keeping his nose vertical) with your left hand towards his right shoulder while your right hand crosses over to lean into his left shoulder stretching his neck. Place your right hand on the right side of his head while your left hand moves across to his right shoulder to stretch his neck to the other side. Turn your right hand so that your fingers point toward his shoulder. Gently press his head from the left side with your left hand (fingers towards his forehead) turning his head onto your right hand (resting on the floor). Exchange directions your hands are pointing and turn his head to the left side.

26. **The Claws.** While his head is still turned to the left, hook your right hand under his occiput (two fingers to each side of his spine). Let his head rest back on your claw which is resting on the floor. Place the claw of your left hand lightly up under his brow, two fingers to each side of his nose. Hold.

27. **The Inch Worm.** Keeping your right claw in his occiput, lay your left hand across his forehead. Hold... Lift his head by raising the heel of your right hand. Lower his head on your fingers which are now raised about an inch up from the occiput. Continue until you have 'inched-wormed' your claw out from under his head (without pulling hair). Lean your right thumb into the crown point on top of his head above the ears.

28. **The Third Eye.** Place the middle finger of your right hand on Small Intestine 19 in front of his right ear (without closing the ear canal). Place the middle finger of your left hand in front of his other ear and, one thumb on top of the other, lean into his third eye.

29. **Over the Eyes.** Place your thumbs to each side of his nose so that you are simultaneously pressing his cheekbones, the inside corners of his eyeballs (lightly) and brow. Repeat on second lines over the middles of his eyeballs. And on third lines over the outside corners of the eyeballs. Apply no pressure to the eyeballs. Do not touch them if his eyes are open or he's wearing contacts.

30. **Under the Cheekbones.** Press Stomach 3 up and under his cheekbones with your middle fingers (on a line down from the middle of the eye).

31. **The Last Large Intestine Points.** Press into Large Intestine 20 to the bottom corners of his nose with your forefingers (without closing the nasal passage).

32. **The Jaw Hinge.** Drop the backs of your fingers down to his chin and, holding it, open and move his chin. Say 'Let your jaw drop'. When it has dropped hold the jaw hinge area pressing lightly into it with the heels of your hands. Hold the temples lightly with both hands until you feel the two sides balance.

33. **The Finish.** Cup your hands over his eyes. Lay your left hand over his third eye and your right over his heart chakra and finish as in Basic.

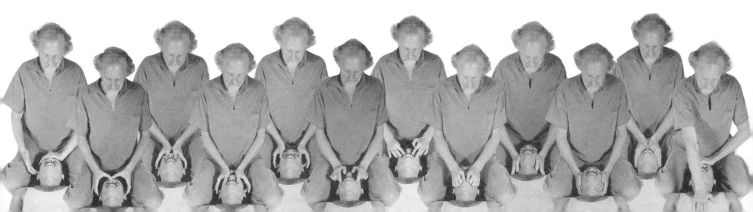

THE HARA

In the following attention is paid to the individual meridians' areas in the Hara (the abdomen). This work, which is very powerful, often puts people into a deep state of peace. It should not be attempted after a meal or, when a person has any inflamation or problem in this area. Masunaga describes working here as stimulating the parasympathetic nervous system. The parasympathetic nervous system is suppressed, shutting down our digestion and other functions not immediately needed when we are faced with danger, and our sympathetic (fight or flight) system takes over; which happens too often in our stressed environment. There is an interesting connection between these two autonomic systems, and tantric lovemaking. It is the para-sympathetic which triggers an erection and the sympathetic which triggers ejaculation. A dominant sympathetic nervous system could be implicated in the two most common forms of male sexual dysfunction; impotency and premature ejaculation. There is no greater enemy of tantra than fear. Another problem of a more mechanical nature, that can cause a man to prematurely ejaculate, is a full bladder. This too can be connected to the sympathetic system which is activated to restrain urination (whereas it is the para-sympathetic which initiates urination).

By stimulating the para-sympathetic nervous system we are helping normalize the body's basic functions. (And the erection men sometimes get during bodywork may have more to do with this and the consequent movement of energy than any lascivious thoughts).

Each of the twelve meridians has its own area in the hara. Go into each area on the outbreath slowly with the fingers and hand relaxed. If you feel a pulse slowly back off. The aorta coming down from the heart should not be pressed into, as there is a danger of its walls being thin.

1. Sitting seiza to the left of the hara, leaning in from your own Hara, do the Basic Co-Centering rocking squeeze.

2. Place your left hand across the hara to mother as the extended fingers of your right hand lean slowly on the outbreath into the following meridian areas, working around the hara in a spiral pattern. The letters designate meridian areas and do not necessarily correspond to the location of the related organs. It will help you remember this pattern to see how the changes in direction your hand makes when working f g h and j k l inscribe the letter H. Do not use any force in the hara, but follow the breath down feeling the letting go in your own hara. While leaning in keep your eyes on the person's face to watch for any reaction.

Lay your hand across his hara just below his navel. With your right hand extended and relaxed so that it bows backward as you lean in, gently lean in with the parts of your fingers just below the tips into the areas related to the following meridians:

    a. Heart (up under sternum)
    b. Stomach (straight down)
    c. Triple heater (under rib cage)
    d. Lung (under rib cage)

Your left hand moves to just above navel to mother over Circulation (e).

Your right hand leans into

    f. Kidney (palm towards illiac crest)
    g. Small Intestine (palm towards crotch)
    h. Large Intestine (palm towards navel)
    i. Bladder (palm towards feet)
    j. Large Intestine (palm towards illiac crest)
    k. Small Intestine (palm towards crotch)
    l. Kidney (palm towards illiac crest)
    m. Spleen (palm towards feet)

Your left hand returns to mother below navel.

Your right hand leans into

    n. Lung (under rib cage)
    o. Liver (under rib cage)
    p. Gall Bladder (under rib cage)
    q. Heart (up under sternum)

Keeping your left hand on his hara, place your right hand on his heart center. Hold.

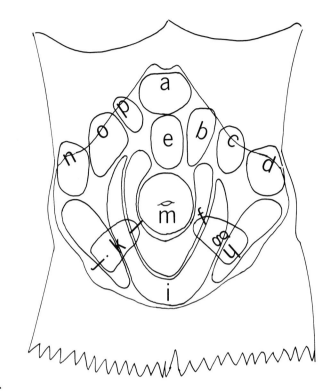

The above areas in the hara relate to the current strength within each meridian. The areas of the back which relate to the holding within each meridian (the more chronic conditions) are mapped below.

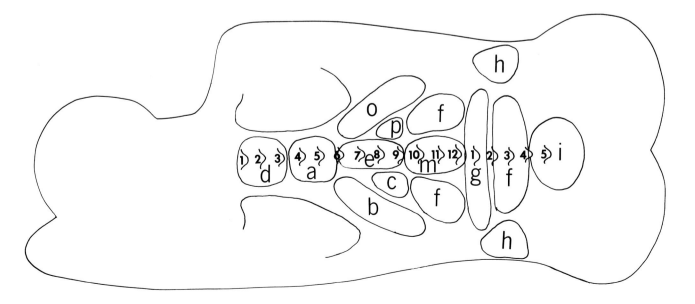

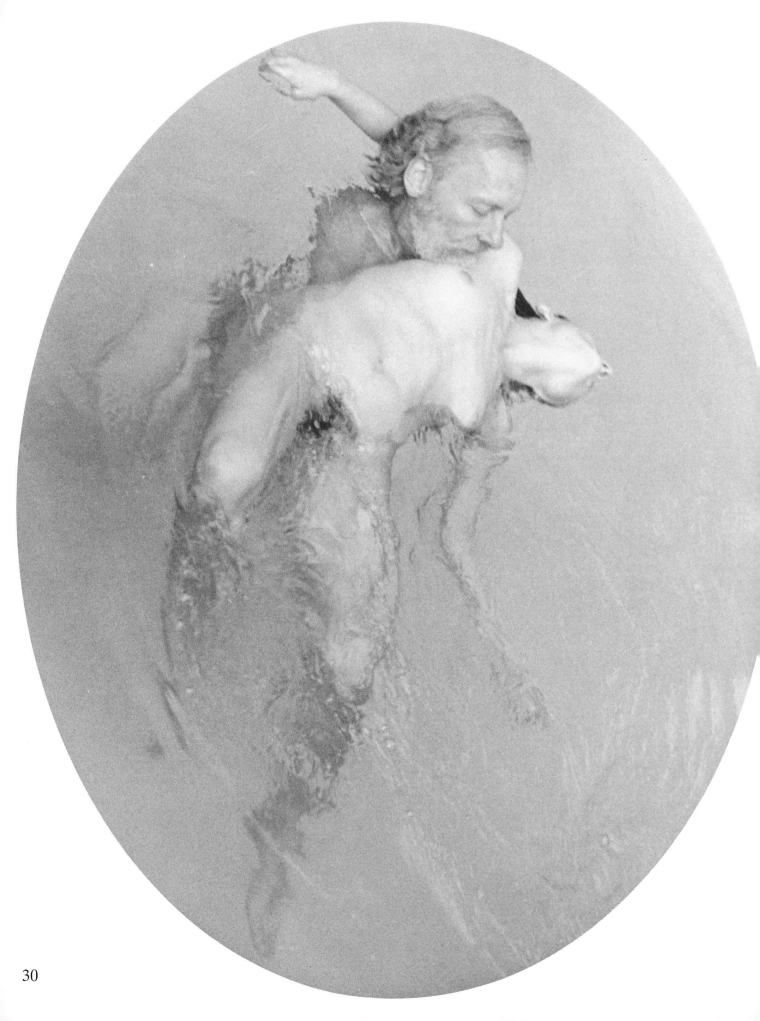

Imagine yourself being floated in a warm pool, the crook of an elbow under your neck, a hand under your sacrum...a gentle rock, a gradual swaying stretching you side to side, a rolling, rolling your spine looser and looser...And while one leg is lifted and rotated your other stretches out as you are swirled through the water...And moments of activity flow into moments of quiet as, held over a shoulder or against a chest or straddling a knee, individual points in arm or back or neck are released.

And after an hour your whole body is more relaxed than it has ever been...energy coursing through every part...And no matter how many feelings you have moved through, whether recollections from the womb, or sorrow that you have not received this kind of nurturing before, at the end you feel completion - energy rising up your back...

Imagine yourself floating someone, feeling their body completely letting go in your arms as you gently rock them, the side of their chest against your chest. You are rocking them with your heart. And as you move them, stretching them, you move them with your heart, so connected do you feel. And as their tension melts away and their spine loosens, in your arms, in their total innocence and trust they become something midway between a child and a lover.

And at the end, when you feel the energy moving up your own back and raise your hand up from their third eye, both your energies intertwine to rise higher and higher...

A Different World

When you step into the water you are in a different world. Bodywork in water is completely different than on land. Differences in size, flexibility and buoyancy from individual to individual are critical in determining what you can or cannot do. The fluidity possible in water make it even clearer than on land that no two sessions can ever be identical. That there is no sequence of moves anyone can do with everyone became obvious when I started the watsu classes here at Harbin. Over the years with the help of students and assistants we have worked out sequences that most people can do with most people. Particularly helpful has been Elaine Marie. Being a foot shorter than me, in the two years she has been learning, practicing and teaching Watsu, she has helped work out solutions to the problems faced when working with people larger than us. The way her, and others who have studied it, make Watsu their own gives testimony to what an open and creative form Watsu is.

It's openness, and the demands for adapting to each person it places on the practicioner, make learning Watsu an excellent training for the bodyworker to develope his creativity, as well as a sense of nurturing connection and flowing movement which, after having studied Watsu, become easier to incorporate in bodywork on land.

In the following 9 lessons differences in size are less important in the first six than in the last three lessons. The first five lessons make up a complete basic Watsu that you should be able to do with almost anybody. But, even with these sequences, it is a good idea, when possible, to first learn them on someone smaller than yourself before practicing them on someone larger. The work on the steps of the sixth lesson can be done with anybody. Most of the moves in the last three lessons are easier when working with someone smaller than you. The sixth, seventh and eighth lessons integrate supportive holding of the first chakra (i.e. having the person straddling your leg while working elsewhere, etc). I have found this connection to be very powerful in assisting the other chakras to open and the energy to rise up the back. In the supportive non-threatening atmosphere of a Watsu, it is particularly effective therapy for those who have fear and tension around intimacy and/or problems from childhood abuse and/or sexual traumatization.

Each of the lessons is to be read first (and visualized) before entering the pool. Feel free to use each lesson as a springboard to practice freestyle, to play and create your own moves.

Preparing Yourself

Rocking. Stand in water that is level with your breasts. Slowly rock from one side to the other (shifting your weight from one leg to the other). Get into a constant rocking that requires no effort and feels good. Feel how, as you rock to one side there is a feeling of movement continuing on past where your body stops. Feel that movement continuing on out from your body each time you rock to each side. Keep your rocking slow enough to feel that movement complete itself to each side before the rock brings you back out the other side. Gradually introduce a sideways rotation into your rock. Feel how the continuation of your turning continues around you and meets the continuation of the turning from the other side to form a circle or a spiral around you. Gradually introduce a freer, dancing movement, as you feel your whole spine loosen and your body become free in its interweaving slowly spiraling web of movement. (this rocking becomes particularly powerful when done with others in a circle.)

Floating in Tonus. Floating with your arms and legs fully extended you can put your whole body into a state of 'tonus,' the state of relaxed strength which we use at many points in Bodywork Tantra(such as when we're leaning in with our arm straight). If you have trouble floating, have someone help you at first, keeping you afloat. Have your arms up over your head, arching your back. First imagine your whole body as rubber - flexible and floppy. Let go in every joint. Nothing is holding you together. Then imagine your whole body as steel - rigid and heavy - tightness in every part. Then imagine yourself as wood, with the strength and flexibility of wood, the life of a tree through your whole body.

When you float on your own, at the beginning keep a deep reservoir of air in your lungs, renewing it from the top with shallow breaths. Keep the whole area around your first chakra as relaxed as possible. Feel the extension out to your fingers and out to your toes. Feel the vibrations up your back as you reach the full extension of your energy, your whole body in a state of tonus.

Once you get used to floating this way, try doing some stretches while floating. Keeping your right leg and arm fully extended, wrap your left arm around your left knee and pull it to your shoulder. Hold. Grab your left foot and pull it out to your left side with your left hand. Hold. Still holding your foot out to your left side, lay your right ankle across your left thigh. Continue floating this way, your right arm still extended up over your head. Slip your right foot underneath your left thigh and hold it with your left hand, stretching it towards your buttock, while floating with your left leg and right arm fully extended. Float with both arms and legs extended and repeat the above to the right side. Float with both knees pulled up to your chest. If you are comfortable in lotus, float in lotus(with practice, by always keeping one arm up above your head, you can bring your legs, one at a time into this position without touching the bottom). The more you practice this the more you will enjoy how free your body can become...and strong. And the more you will be able to use this strength of 'tonus' in your work.

Preparing the Place

To do watsu you need a pool large enough to move a person around in. You should have at least ten feet to rock them back and forth. The ideal depth for you to work in is water level with your breasts. A wall to lean back against and steps to sit with someone on will allow a wider range of possible moves. The ideal temperature is around 93 degrees Fahrenheit. Much over that and you will overheat while working. Under 88 degrees the person receiving will begin to get cold. If you work in a cooler pool keep sessions short.

Preparing the Person

Before working on anyone find out if he has any problems or conditions that could be worsened by stretching, pressure, movement or hot water. Find out if he has any problems with his neck or back. Be sure to keep his neck supported throughout without letting the head fall back. Tell him to let you know if anything is uncomfortable, if he feels too cold, or if he is overheating (at which point you should stop).

Stand to the persons right. Place the crook of your left arm behind his neck and lay him back into a floating position raising him with your right hand under his sacrum. His left arm is behind your back. (The above, and what follows, can be reversed if you are left handed). Hold still in the water feeling him float without moving in your arms. If he is a 'sinker' and he feels heavy in your arms, slip your right forearm under the backs of his knees and bend his knees up (letting him sink lower) just far enough to feel his weight equally distributed between your two arms. Begin slowly rocking him in that position, establishing a 'basic rock', before slipping your right hand back under his sacrum and continuing as follows.

1. **The Basic Rock.** Slowly start to rock him. If the water's level allows you to spread your legs, rock from one leg to the other. Do not try to force the person to stay all the way up on the surface if he tends to sink. If his legs are heavy you can brace your right elbow on the side of your hip to support him. Your goal is to find the most comfortable position within which you can abandon yourself into a steady hypnotic rocking.

Rock and rock holding the side of his chest against the front of your chest (your heart center). Feel how you are holding and rocking him with your heart. Feel how open your heart is. After this basic rock becomes completely automatic and timeless, feel whatever other movements gradually grow out of it. Flow slowly into them. You may find your body leaning into his waist and your hand pulling him back to rock him laterally. You might lower yourself into the water as your arms lift his opposite side, and then stand high as his opposite side lowers. Repeating this can create a rhythmic rolling.

Return as often as it feels natural to the Basic Rock. Try resting the side of your head (face towards his feet) on his heart center at the same time as you rock him.

Each time continue the Basic Rock until the next movement grows naturally out of it. As you do this with more people you will find that each has his own basic rock.

2. **Knees Up Rock.** While rocking the person towards his head let your right forearm slip down under the backs of his knees. Rock him with your forearm under his knees.

Then bring his knees up towards his chest. If possible bring his head onto your chest and hold him close to your heart. Gently rock him.

A Simple Finish. *If you are in a pool with a wall, back up to the wall holding him with his knees up. Lean back against the wall, your left leg straight, and raise your right knee propping your right foot on your left leg. Let the backs of his legs rest on your raised right thigh. While his head is resting on your heart center, stroke his face gently with your right hand. Hold his third eye with your middle finger (your left hand can be holding his heart center at the same time). As you feel the movement up your own back, raise your right hand high into the air and lower it into the water. Hold him still for a moment and then slowly lower your right leg standing him on his feet. Let him lean against you for a while. If you have someone who is not ready to stand on his own you can place his hands on a railing (if one is available) and/or say something to reassure him that it is O.K. to come back, etc. If steps are available you can finish sitting on the steps with him instead of backing up to a wall.*

Begin with the Basic Rock and the knees up rock of Lesson I. Hold him close to your chest, his knees up, and feel his breathing. Connect to his breathing.

3. **The Accordian.** As he breathes in slowly open your arms. When ready to breathe out close your arms bringing his knees back up to his chest. Continue opening and closing with the breathing. Each time you spread your arms feel the opening of your own chest.

4. **The Rotating Accordian.** Continue as above. As you open and close your arms inscribe a circle in the air with his knees on a plane parallel to the water's surface. In order to add some stretching to this rotation you can brace his hips against your side. Keep it slow. Do not let this, or any move, build up to a frenetic or dizzying pace.

5. **The Near Leg Rotation**. Continue rotating the two knees as above. Rotate his knees in a clockwise direction. While bringing them up and towards you let his far leg slip off your arm. Continue rotating the near leg by itself.

Start turning your body in a clockwise direction so that the resistance of the water stretches the far leg while you continue to rotate the near leg.

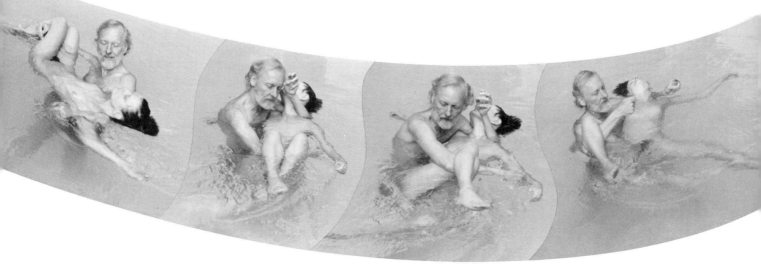

6. **Far Leg Rotation.** Slip the crook of your right elbow under his far leg and rotate it. As with all your movements do this as much as possible with your whole body, and not just your arm, moving his whole body through the water. If, in the process, his chest comes up flat across your chest, hold it there for a moment. Continue, getting freer in your movements (without speeding them up). If easily accessible, you might hold and work for a moment his left shoulder with your right hand (your right arm still under his knee).

Slip your right hand back under his sacrum and return to the Basic Rock. Repeat the knees up rock and finish with the simple finish of Lesson I.

Optional Arm/Knee Locks. If you have someone flexible and your arm under his knee(s) can comfortably reach his upper arm, try, when you have either or both knees up to his chest during the above rotations, pulling the crook of his elbow under the back of his knee(s). Holding his left wrist (his arm locked under his knee(s) with your right hand and his neck and occiput with your left hand float him out away from you. Letting his right arm slip out in front of you, rock and slowly move him through the water. Move behind him resting his head on your shoulder. Experiment and play with the possibilities these arm/leg(s) locks offer.

Begin with the sequences of Lesson I and II.

7. **Far Leg Over.** Rotate the far leg with your right arm, the crook of your left elbow still under his neck. Hold his left ankle and, bending his knee, lift his leg up over your head and drop the back of his left knee across your shoulder. If you feel any pressure against your throat turn your head towards his feet. While lifting his leg pay special attention to his head, making sure his nose doesn't go under. If he feels heavy on your shoulder lower yourself into the water spreading and/or bending your knees.

Once comfortable, with your left arm still under his neck, hold his upper back with your left hand and with your right hand reach up his back as far as you can comfortably and press your fingers into the line of points that parallel the spine (the Bladder meridian on the side away from the water), working down, alongside the back, on the sacrum, the buttock and the top of the leg.

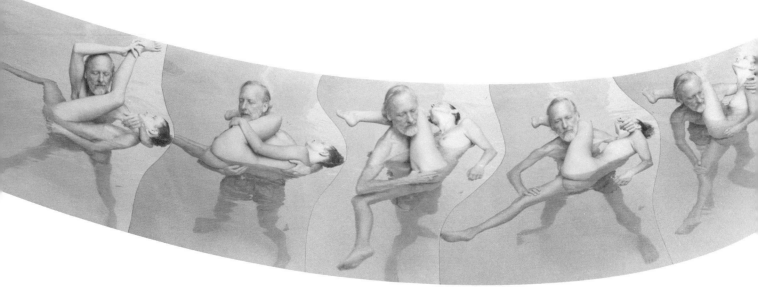

8. **The Leg Push.** With your right hand holding his right leg above his knee push the leg away from you. While pushing his leg away, turn in a clockwise direction so that the water's resistance adds to the push, stretching the far leg further.

9. **The Leg Around the Waist.** Keeping the crook of your left elbow under his neck, continue pushing his right leg away from you. Push it towards the bottom. Stepping around it bring his right leg up around the left side of your waist. With your left arm pull his upper body as close to your left shoulder as possible.

Holding him close with your left arm, hook the fingers of your right hand into the top of the sacrum and pull down, stretching the spine.

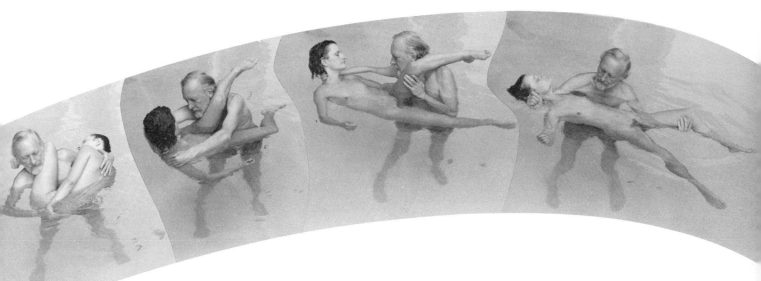

10. **The Leg off To The Second Side.** Making sure his left arm is floating out to his side so that it will end up behind your back, reach up with your right hand and hold the back of his neck. Once you have a good hold of his neck with your right hand, take your left arm out from under it. Lower yourself into the water so that his left leg slips off your shoulder.

Hold his sacrum with your left hand and slip the crook of your right elbow under his neck (his left arm should be behind your back).

Begin rocking him from his left side (Since you have your right arm under his neck you can start out by paying special attention to working and stretching the neck). Continue with the mirror image of moves 1-10. When you return to his right side bring his knees back up and go on to the simple finish.

Do the sequences of I-III and their mirror image returning to the side and position you started from. Repeat the near leg rotation.

11. **The Near Leg Over.** While rotating the near leg pick it up at the ankle and slip the back of the right knee over your left shoulder. Keeping the crook of your left elbow (or your hand) under his neck, stretch the far leg out with your right hand as you turn clockwise. Rock his far leg, pushing and rolling his thigh with your right hand.

12. **The Leg Under and Across.** Dip lower in the water and bring him to a vertical position by simultaneously swinging up his upper body and pressing down his left leg. With his right leg still over your shoulder and his left leg straight and braced against the inside of your right leg, work down along both sides of his spine with the fingers of both hands (his head resting on his right knee). Reaching over his left arm, hold his neck in the crook of your right elbow. Keep his right leg on your shoulder as you push his left leg across and in front of you so that it floats out to your left. Hold his shoulder with one hand as the other squeezes and works down his right arm. Stretch and work his right hand.

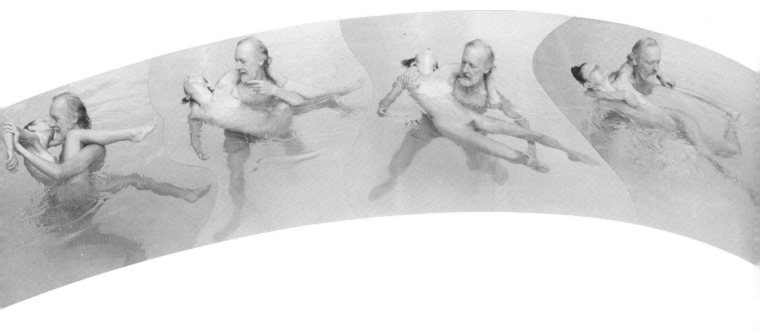

13. **The Twist.** Hold his neck with your left hand as your right arm comes out from under his neck and slips under his left arm. Hold his neck with your right hand. Dip your right shoulder under his left shoulder. Lower your left shoulder into the water so that his right leg slips off. Catching it in the crook of your left elbow, keep it bent and pulled across his other leg as your right hand (your right arm still under his left shoulder) pulls down his right shoulder, twist stretching his spine.

14. **The Leg Under.** Release his right leg, and, quickly slipping your left hand under his left leg, catch his right ankle before his right leg straightens. Move him through the water pulling his right foot, being careful to keep his neck supported. Work the bottom of his foot. Release the ankle and, supporting his neck with your right hand, move him freely through the water.

Slip the crook of your elbow under his neck (his left arm behind you), rotate the near leg, and, bringing it over your shoulder, work a mirror image of the above. Afterwards, both his knees up, bring him to the wall for the simple finish.

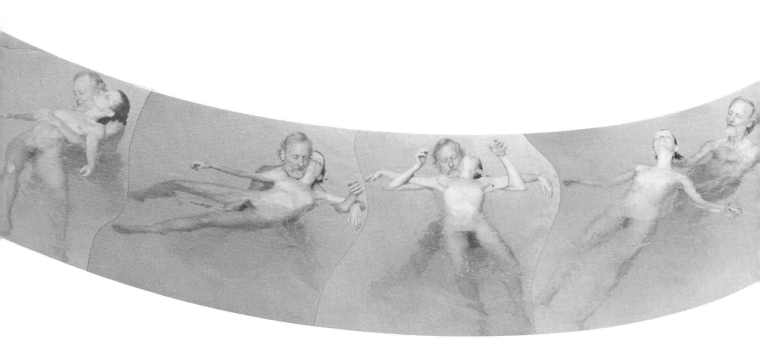

Repeat the sequences of lessons I-IV. If you want to shorten the sequence the following can be inserted after Lesson III's 'leg off to the second side' by coming out to the side with his arm in front of you. If you have done IV, you can pull his arm that is over your shoulder up and slip out...

15. **From Above the Head.** Move up to above his head, placing his head on your left shoulder. Hold his buttocks (or lower back) with both hands and move him through the water, rocking him. You can work the back stretching and working up it with both hands (avoid arching it too far back). You can reach under his arms and, holding his occiput, lift his head to stretch his neck. You can also work with his arms from this position, spreading them wide and/or crossing them as you move backwards through the water.

16. **Knees Up From Above.** There are three ways to pull his knees to his chest while behind him.

a) If your arms are long enough, you can reach his knees from behind and pull them up.

b) While behind him you can float him slowly towards a wall so that his feet butting the wall bend his knees to within your reach.

c) A method used by Elaine Marie is to cross his arms and press his hands to the sides of his chest. Then as you keep him wrapped up in his self hug, you move to his side. Bring both knees up and, keeping hold of them, return to above his head.

Once you have his knees pulled up to his chest you can move him through the water and then back up to either the wall or the steps.

17. **Knees Up Finish.** You can either finish on the wall or on the steps.

a) Back up to the wall. Pull his knees even closer to his chest. Hold. Place your left knee under him propped on your right leg. Lower him onto your knee, making sure his neck is comfortable on your shoulder and not bent too far back. Reach under his shoulders with both hands and pull his chest open. Hold. Place one hand on his heart center and one hand on his body center, just below the navel. Hold. Leave your left hand where it is and slipping your hand out lift it out of the water and flick any excess water off your fingers. With your middle finger slide up the front of his nose to his third eye. Hold, feeling the connection between the center your left hand is on and the third eye. Hold. Feel the energy moving up your own spine. Slowly lift both hands off raising your right up and then lowering it into the water. Hold his hands from underneath lightly touching the center of his palms with your middle fingers. Slowly lower his feet to the ground, lowering your knee. Let him lean against you until he's ready to stand on his own feet. (This finish is illustrated by the last four moves at the bottom of page 49.)

If you are working with someone larger than you, you may need to lower his feet to the floor right after the knees up stretch. Or, if steps are available you might find it more comfortable to finish on the steps as follows.

b) Back up to the steps, floating him from behind, his knees up. Sit on the steps with him between your legs. At this point you can do additional work on his face, etc. (His head is still resting comfortably on your left shoulder.) Pull his chest open with both hands. Place one on the body center and one on the heart center. Hold. After flicking the water off your right hand, slide your middle finger up the front of his nose to his third eye and hold. Lift both hands off to finish.

LESSON VI Stepwork

This lesson presents a sequence which can be done with someone sitting on steps. It can be incorporated in either the previous sequence or the sequence which follows. If there are no steps where you are working proceed to Lesson VII. Ideal steps would be in a corner of a pool with walls to each side of the steps to lean back against. Begin as in Lesson I with the Basic and the knees up rock.

1. **The Step Positioning.** Keeping his knees held up to his chest, back up to and sit on the steps. If there is a wall alongside the steps, sit sideways, your back to the wall, his right arm still behind you(under where your back contacts the wall). Make sure his right elbow is not caught on the next step up. You should be high enough up on the steps so that you can lay his head on your chest, on your heart center. Pull both knees even tighter into his chest. Let go of them and, before his left leg straightens, slip your right arm under his left knee and pull it up to his chest. Hold it there and wrap your right leg around his right leg, your foot under him on the next step down from the one you're sitting on. Let go of his left leg and slip it past your right knee. He is now straddling your right calf(your left foot is on the same step you're sitting on, your left leg against his back). Hold his head to your heart center with both hands.

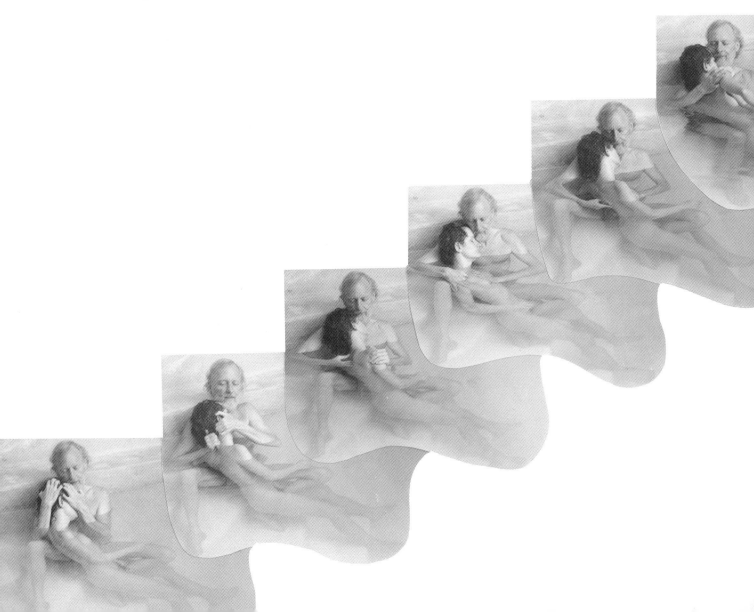

2. **Stepwork.** Work the face freestyle (or as in the tantsu side position)... Work the head...the back of the neck...the top of the shoulder...around the shoulder blade...and across the front of the chest. Hold the heart center with your right hand and work down alongside the spine with your left thumb. Rotate the shoulder. Work out the arm and hand. Rotate and stretch his arm. Lay his arm up behind his head. Work down his side. Work the lower back and left buttock. Pull his left leg up (if easy to reach you can stretch, rotate and work on his left foot, here). Slip your right leg out from around his right leg, letting him float up on his back. You can, at this point, support his sacrum with your right knee, prop his head on a step, or on your left knee, and work his hara.

Slip his arm back behind your back and return into the middle of the pool to continue the Basic sequence. When you arrive at his second side, bring his knees up, float him to the other side of the steps and work a mirror image of the above (all except the Hara work).

3. **The Step Rock.** Bring his left arm in front of you and float him out so that both your knees (your feet on a step) are in his lower back. Hold his head by the occiput. Gently move and rotate his head at the same time as your knees rock him (keeping your toes on a step and rhythmically lifting your heels).

Float him out to work in the middle and/or bring his knees up and finish against the wall, etc.

LESSON VII The Gyroscope

This lesson, and the next, work best with someone not too large to handle. To make a complete sequence incorporating this, begin with the basic rock, the knees up rock, the stepwork (on the near side), the accordian, the rotating accordian, and the near leg rotation. Pull the near leg through the water so that the water's resistance stretches the far leg.

1. The Gyroscope. Reach over the near leg with your right arm and clasp it to your side, your right hand holding his right buttock. Continue moving him through the water with his thigh clasped to your side. Moving with your whole body, lower his clasped leg lower into the water at the same time as his upper body slowly rises forward and up. Keeping your arm under his neck let his upper back slowly fall back. Continue doing this giving him each time a sense of a gyroscoping slow free fall back into the water, his upper body transcribing a counter-clockwise circle.

2. The Sacral Rock. Your right hand lets go of the buttock and hooks its four fingers into the top of the sacrum (the flat plate at the base of the spine). Hold him for a moment to your chest, pulling down on his sacrum. Roll him back out flat in the water and pull rocking him towards his feet and, with the crook of your elbow under his neck, rock him back towards his head. Continue rocking him, stretching his spine.

3. The Leg Hold. With the crook of your left elbow under his neck and his right arm behind your back, rotate his far leg with your right arm (as in lesson II). Notice how freely his other leg can move through the water. Move his right foot towards the bottom and clasp his right thigh between your thighs. Continue rotating his far leg, stretching it.

4. Moving Between the Legs. With your right arm still under his left knee, reach up with your right hand and grasp his upper arm. Hold his neck with your left hand. Move your left leg to the inside of his right leg, both your legs now between his legs. Still holding under his left knee, turn sideways and float him up to straddle your left hip.

5. The Body Pull. Still holding his neck and occiput, reach down with your right hand and push his left leg away from you. Rock it gently. Work down the back of the calf between the muscles with your thumb. Hold and pull his left foot (or his leg), stretching the whole body. Press his foot up towards his left buttock. Work the bottom of his foot. Keep supporting his neck and, facing him, work his back with your right hand. Replace your left hand under his neck with your right and, turning sideways, work his right leg and foot as above.

6. The Roll Over. Without letting go of his foot (still pressed towards his buttock) or his neck (not letting his head fall back), bring his upper body up and over, his chest landing on your chest.

You can roll him back onto his back and finish from this side.

You have just finished the last lesson, rolling your Watsu partner up onto your chest.

7. **The Back Hold.** Still holding his right foot, back up to the wall so that his left leg is to the inside of your right leg. Wrap your left leg around his left leg and prop your left foot (or leg) on your right knee (your right leg is straight). Let go of his right foot so that he settles straddling your left thigh.

His chest is against your chest (Make sure his head and neck are comfortable and that there is no skin or breast pull where the chests contact). With your arms under his arms, work down alongside the spine (the Bladder meridian), pressing your fingers in with each outbreath. Continue down the sacrum, and finish holding to each side of the tail bone.

8. **Shoulder and Arm Work.** Hold his right shoulder with your left hand and work around the blade with your right thumb. Rotate his shoulder with both hands. Pull his right arm back and work with both hands. Work and stretch his wrist and fingers.

9. **The Twist.** With your left hand bring his right arm in front of him (between your chests). Hold it at the wrist with your right hand and keep pulling it across as your left hand reaches up and pulls his left shoulder back, stretch twisting his spine (keeping it as straight vertically as possible). While he is still twisted out work his left shoulder and arm with both hands. Pull his left arm across his front, pulling his right shoulder back with your right hand. If his right leg feels like its about to slip around and off your knee, reach down with your left hand and pull it, letting go of his left arm, to continue twist stretching him. Holding his right knee with your left hand, slip your leg out from under him. Bring his right knee up to his chest. Hold it there with your right hand as your left hand brings up his left knee.

10. **The Neck Lift**. With your back to the wall, his back on your chest, pull both his knees into his chest. (Your arms under his arms). Reach your hands up under his occiput and lift standing straight, stretching his neck. While still holding him up, bend your left knee in front of you, propping your left foot against your right leg (which is straight). Lower him so that he is straddling your left thigh.

11. **Chin Work.** Still holding under his occiput with your thumbs, lean your chin into his right shoulder between his neck and scapula. Hold with your chin while your right thumb works down the right side of his neck (alongside the spine). Your left thumb is still in the occiput. Hold the occiput with both thumbs, move your chin to his left shoulder and work down the neck with your left thumb.

12. **Face Work**. Holding the occiput with both thumbs again, prop the back of his head against your third eye. Work freestyle on his face with your fingers, working his jaw open, etc. Hold both hands cupped over his eyes shutting out all outside light. Hold... Lift him and reset him far enough out on your leg to be able to lay his head back on your left shoulder comfortably.

Finish as in lesson V.

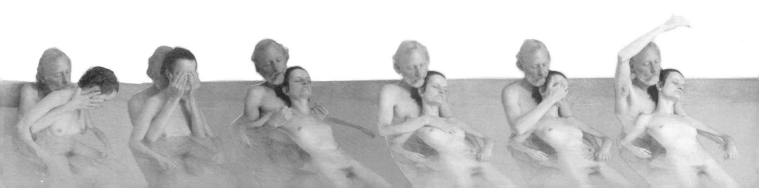

LESSON IX Freestyle

If you have learned the moves and sequences of the first 8 lessons, you probably already know more moves than you could put into any one session... And you have probably found out how important it is to have a variety of moves, a repetoire to draw from to match the variety of sizes and shapes of people you might find yourself floating in the water. And by now you probably have realized that these moves can be put together in any order or combinations that works as long as you keep the neck supported, the nose up out of the water and the back unstrained, etc. Now you are ready to develop your own ways of putting these together...and your own moves. Some of the range of possibilities not included so far in these lessons are illustrated here. Make up your own. Play is divine.

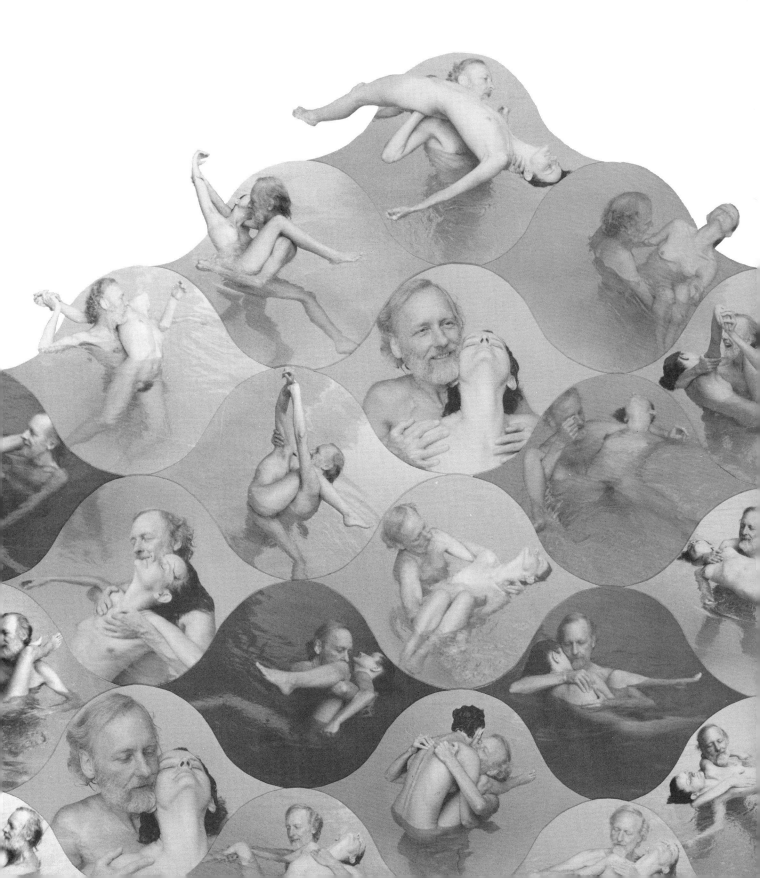

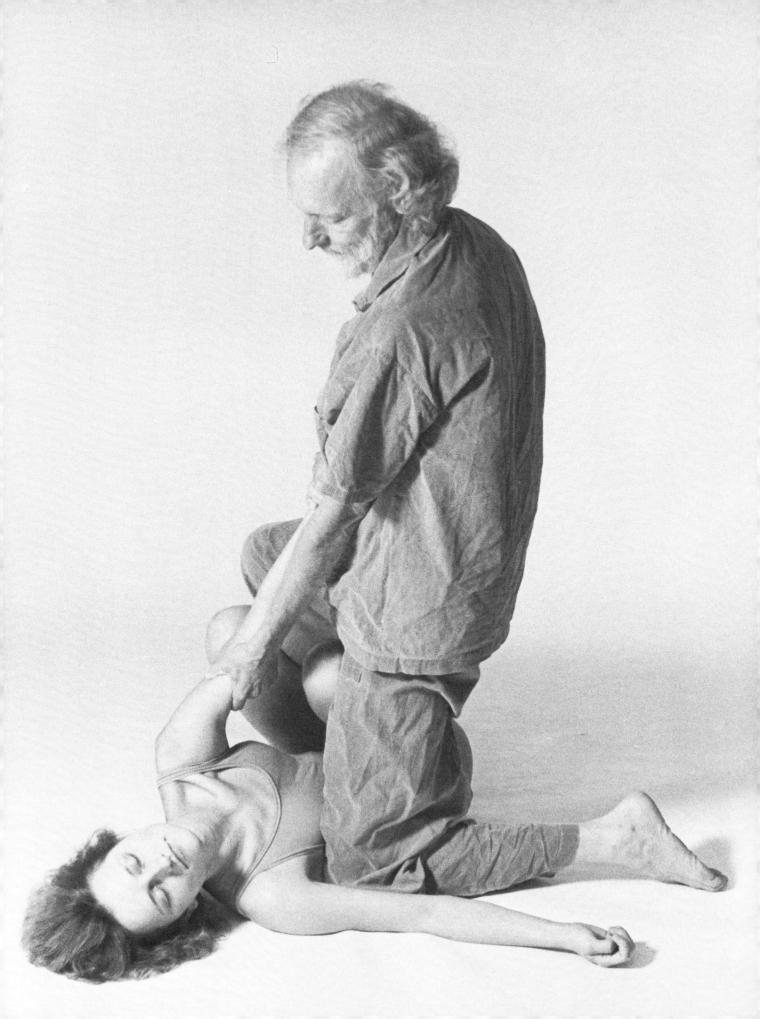

In Co-centering you learn to use your body to lean in with as you feel your connection to someone in your own hara. In Watsu, you learn to feel that connection in your heart center, and to move someone from that center aided by the water's nurturing support and the freedom of movement it allows. In Tantsu you use your whole body, and a connection with your chakras, to provide that nurturing support. In many of Tantsu's moves you cradle and enfold someone as you lean into your own hara. The greater you feel this, and the greater you feel your heart open, the greater you will feel the rising up your own back as you lift your hands off the person's heart center and third eye at the end.

It is this sense of spiritual intimacy which gives Tantsu its power.

In what follows you will learn simple patterns in four basic Tantsu positions. The first two positions combine easily with Co-centering.

You will be working on the floor to cradle someone. At least half the time you will be sitting in what I call side straddle, that is with one foot in front of you and one out to your side. If you are not used to these positions, it may take some time to get comfortable with them. Practice sitting and gently moving and stretching in side-straddle before working in them. You can place a cushion under the hip that is on the side you are straddled toward. If necessary you can straighten out the leg that is bent out to the side. If you begin feeling pain do not stay in this position. You will find using the side straddle gradually opens your hips and increases your flexibility.

The Side

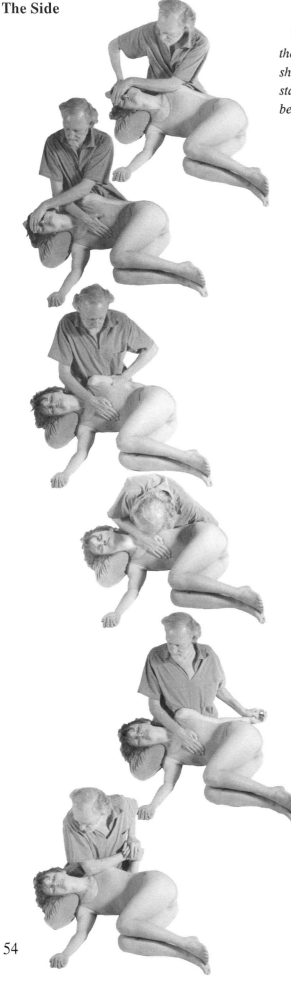

For most people, lying on their side is their most comfortable position, the one they choose for sleeping. It is the best position for working on the shoulder and the meridian of the side, the Gall Bladder. While the person stays in one position on their side, we work from three positions -- 1. From behind their back, 2. From above their head, 3. From below their hips.

Your Tantsu partner is on his right side. His legs pulled up into a foetal position in front of him. Have a rolled up towel or cushion nearby to slip under his head. Sit side straddle behind his back, your left foot in front of you and your right leg bent out to the side. Your left toes should be level with the top of his right shoulder, your left knee touching his back. Sit as close to your left heel as possible.

1. **The Head Hold.** Simultaneously pick up his left forearm with your left hand and his head with your right hand. While pulling his left arm and lifting his head, slide your right thigh under his head right up against his shoulders. Lay his left arm comfortably across your left leg and his neck over your right thigh. Making sure his neck is completely supported by your leg and his head is not turned to either side, hold the top of his head (his crown chakra) with your right hand and place your left hand across his forehead centered on his third eye. Hold feeling the connection between these two chakras (your own back should be as straight as is comfortable).

2. **Heart and Mind.** Still holding his forehead with your left hand, reach under your left arm with your right hand and place it on his heart chakra (be sure there is no pressure on his throat). Hold, feeling the connection between these two chakras, your own back straight.

3. **Squeeze out Arm.** Keeping your right hand on the heart chakra, clasp his upper arm with your left hand, and, on an outbreath, lean over it and squeeze, feeling that you are taking it into your own hara. On each subsequent outbreath lean over and squeeze into a place further out his left arm.

4. **Circulation Point.** When you reach his hand hold the point in the center of his palm with your thumb (Be careful not to bend his arm backward at elbow). Feel the connection between this point and the heart chakra.

5. **The Triangle.** Keeping his left elbow on your leg, swing his lower arm up with your left hand at the same time as your right hand lifts off his heart chakra and holds his left arm just below the wrist (your right forearm resting across his upper chest just below his shoulder) making a triangle (his arm and your forearm). Bend his hand back and forth with your left hand.

6. **Arm Rotation.** Lift his arm up with your left hand (at his wrist) and press his arm to your chest with your right arm. (His hand is to the left of your head). Lean back gently to stretch. Rotate in both directions.

7. **Stretch to Second side.** Switching his wrist into your right hand move his arm to the right side of your neck. Press it to your chest with your left arm and lean back to stretch. Lay his arm out up over his head.

8. **Leg Pull.** Slip your hands around his left thigh and lean back to pull (Keep his leg close to his side). Lower his leg. At the same time reach under and pull his right leg closer to his chest so that both legs are bent up as far as possible into a foetal position.

9. **The Rest.** With your right forearm gently slide his left arm back out in front of him. Either let his head stay resting on your right thigh or let it slip off in front of it, whichever looks more comfortable. With both arms circle and gently press his shoulder and tailbone while resting the side of your head on the side of his hip and letting your chest rest against his side. Feel the opening in your own heart center as you lie there.

10. **Above the Head.** Get up on your knees. Place your left hand on the floor and, holding his head in your right hand, slide your left knee up to behind his shoulder. Switch his head into your left hand and, placing your right hand on the floor, slide your right knee out in front of him. Sit side straddle with your right foot in front of you and lower his head onto your thigh (his ear between your thigh and your calf), the back of his head against your hara, your left knee against his upper back. Moving into this second position you have reversed the configuration of your knees without lifting them off the floor. Be sure that you are well above him so that his neck continues the natural foetal curve and is not bent back.

11. **Occiput-Third Eye.** Hold the large depressions (GB20) under his occiputal ridge to each side of the neck with your left thumb and forefinger. Hold his third eye (just above his nose) with your right middle finger.

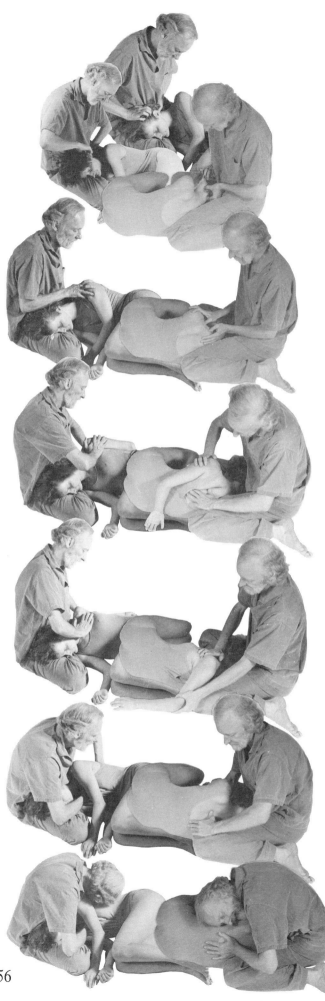

12. **Small Intestine Point.** Keeping thumb and finger in the occiput, place the middle finger of your right hand in the depression (Small Intestine 19) in front of the ear opening (do not close the ear canal).

13. **The Side of Head.** Your Thumb and fingers still in the occiput, work gently up the temple in front of the ear. Work the skull around and behind the ear, holding whatever indentations your fingers slip into. When they arrive at the occiput, replace your left thumb with your right middle finger.

14. **The Neck Squeeze.** Maintaining your finger hooked under the occiput, work down the back of his neck with your left hand, thumb and fingers squeezing between each vertebra. Repeat two more times.

15. **G.B.21.** Place your left thumb in Gall Bladder 21 just to the back of his shoulder, just out from the base of the neck. Hold (your finger still hooked under the occiput).

16. **Top of Shoulder.** Keep leaning into G.B. 21 with your left thumb as your right thumb leans into three places out the top of his shoulder.

17. **The Shoulder Blade.** Still holding G.B. 21, pick up his left arm with your right hand and slip it bent behind his back. With your right hand slide his shoulder up and towards his front. Place your left thumb just under the upper corner of his shoulder blade. As he breathes out gently slide his blade over your thumb (brace your arm with your left elbow on your left thigh). As he breathes in pull his shoulder up again and move your thumb an inch or so down the edge of the blade. On the next out-breath slide the blade back over your thumb. Repeat until you arrive at the bottom of the shoulder blade

18. **Across Chest.** With your left hand pull his upper left arm back as your right fingers work across his upper chest (between the ribs). Place your right hand on his heart chakra.

19. **Upper Back.** Lay his left arm back out in front. Keeping your right hand on his chest, work down upper back starting just below his neck. On each outbreath lean into the next point down feeling its connection into the heart chakra your right hand continues to hold. These points are about an inch to the left of the midline of the spine between each pair of vertebras. Work down until you feel your thumb leaning into a point directly behind the heart chakra.

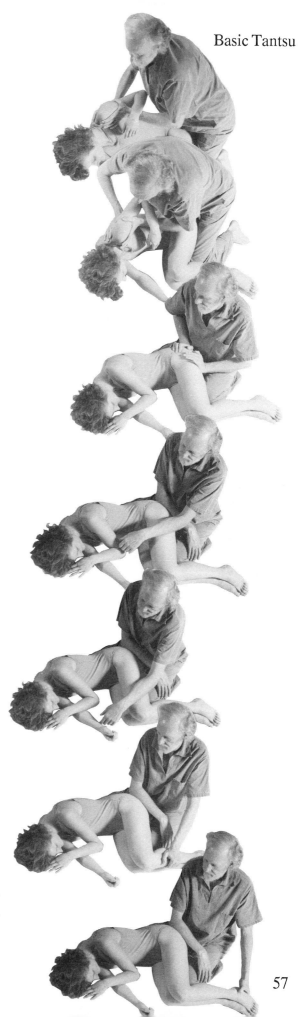

20. **The Heart Hold.** With your whole hand press his spine feeling the connection to your hand on the heart chakra. If you want you can rest your head (facing behind him) on the side of his chest. Lift his head with your left hand. As you slide out from under slip the rolled up towel or cushion under his head.

21. **The Shoulder Rotation.** Pick up his left arm at the wrist with your right hand and take it with you as you move into the third position below him. Up on your knees, straddle his thighs and lower back. Drape his left wrist over your left arm and clasp his left shoulder with both hands (Do not interlace your fingers). Keep his left elbow bent between your two arms and his shoulder firmly clasped between the heels of both hands as you rotate and gently stretch it to all directions. Lay left arm out in front of him.

22. **The Hip Rotation.** Sit back on your heels. Hold his left buttock with both hands and slowly rotate. Change direction. Hold it lightly and rotate faster. Change direction. Keeping hands where they are, vibrate. Hold.

23. **Down Side of Leg.** Lean your right forearm into the depression over the hip joint (GB 30) as your left forearm gently leans in on the outbreath into three more places down the outside of the left thigh. Continue down the side of the calf with the heel of your left hand. With your left thumb hold GB 40 in the indentation just below and to the front of the ankle as you still lean into the hip joint.

24. **Knees up.** Lay his left arm out behind him. Stand and bring both his knees up and, straddling them, press them towards his chest while keeping his sacrum flat on the floor (lean in just below his knees). Keeping his legs bent up, roll him onto his left side and work a mirror image of the above. When you have finished his second side, roll him onto his back and, straightening his legs and neck (his arms out to the side), sit seiza to the right of his hara. Cross your left hand onto his hara just below his navel at the same time as you place your right hand on his heart chakra. Hold...

To combine Tantsu Sides with Co-centering

Do the face down Co-centering. When you roll the person onto his back, instead of sitting beside his hara, stand and, first tucking his pants legs up, press his knees down and roll him to the right, keeping him in a foetal position. Work both sides. Roll him onto his back; sit beside his hara and do the face up Co-centering (The work out the arms can be left out).

The Leg Cradle

In the following you cradle the whole leg in your lap and maintain contact with the first two chakras as you work foot and leg. When you hold a person so completely and in so many places it becomes easier for them to surrender because they no longer know where to resist. This is a powerful position for opening up the Yin meridians in the leg and working up energy into the hara. Use this to open a complete Tantsu or end a session combining Co-centering and Tantsu. Sit seiza alongside your Tantsu partner's hara (hara to hara). Center yourself. Look at his breathing.

1. **Hara-Heart.** Simultaneously lay your left hand across his hara (just below the navel) and your right hand on his heart chakra. Hold...connect to his breathing....

2. **The Top Of The Thighs.** Keep your left hand on his hara. Without changing your position, reach across him (your elbow crooked out) and lean into the top of his thigh with the heel of your right hand (your fingers pointed outwards) as he breathes out. Keeping your forearm vertical, lean into the middle of his thigh, and into the thigh just above the knee. Maintaining your position alongside his hara, lean into the top of the near thigh (fingers pointed upward), into the middle of the thigh (fingers pointed toward the opposite leg), and just above the knee.

3. **The Leg Wrap.** Still sitting alongside his hara, raise his right knee until his foot is flat on the floor. Tuck his pants up to allow stretching. Holding his knee from the outside, continue raising it until his leg (bent) reaches the point where it requires no effort to hold it up. Keeping his leg balanced get up on both knees and place your right knee on the floor against his first chakra (the perineum where it will stay throughout the whole sequence) and your left knee against the outside of his hip. Your left hand still on his hara, bring your left shoulder level with his raised knee. Clasp his bent leg to your chest. Hold it like a baby.

4. **The Outward Leg Rotation.** With your body lean his right leg towards his chest slowly stretching it. (You can, at this point, if possible, rest your forehead on his heart chakra.) Rotate his leg in a direction up to and away from his chest (without letting your hand on the Hara press into the rib cage).

5. **The Foot Rotation.** Carry the rotation into the foot, letting his leg slip under your shoulder across your lap. Hold his ankle with thumb and finger (Kidney 6 and Bladder 62) and the bottom of his foot with your forearm as your body continues to roll.

6. **The Foot Bottom.** With your elbow crooked out press your right thumb into Kidney 1 in the bottom of the foot. Hold. Press three or four more places in a clockwise circle around the softer part of the sole returning to Kidney 1. Hold.

7. **The Foot Forward Stretch.** Hooking his heel on the side of your right leg, press the top of his foot forward.

8. **The Foot Squeeze.** Clasp the foot just below the toes with a vise like grip, the heel of your right hand pressing the side below the big toe and your right fingers pressing the other side. Release and clasp working your way down the foot, around the heel and onto the Achilles tendon.

9. **Spleen.** With your right thumb work up the inside of the calf, just under the bone, leaning in on each outbreath (Spleen 6, 7 ,8 and 9).

10. **Liver Stretch.** Keep your hand on his hara. Place your right hand on the inside of his thigh just above his right knee. Raise up on your knees. Work the Liver meridian up the inside of his thigh leaning into three or four places with the heel of your right hand (keeping your arms straight and your left knee just far enough away from his hip to allow his leg to stretch down.

11. **Knee Press.** Take your hand off his hara and swing his right knee toward his chest. Stand, lifting the other knee with your right hand. Holding his legs just below the knees (at Stomach 36), press both knees keeping his sacrum flat on the floor.

12. **The Shoulder Rock.** Hold his bent legs between your legs. Drop your butt and, keeping your back straight, drop your arms, hooking your fingers around the backs of his shoulders. Rock back (without raising his head off the floor). Rock slowly just rocking your weight (without straining your back). Rock back, alternate hands pulling. Straighten his neck. Lean into the upper corners of his chest (Lung 1 and 2).

13. **The Second Leg.** Lower the leg you have already worked on. Get down on both knees, positioning them against his perineum and his hip. Clasp his left leg to your chest and work a mirror image of above.

To combine the leg cradle with co-centering, begin with the Face Down Co-Centering. Do both sides Tantsu. Then roll him onto his back, do the Hara work and continue with the Leg Cradle. After the second leg, press his knees back up towards his chest and continue with the Basic Co-Centering pattern on to the finish.

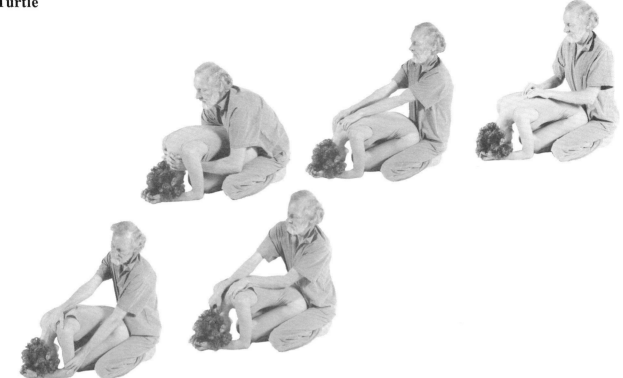

Earlier in this book the problem some people have lying face down on the floor was mentioned. An alternate position to work on the back can be used in Tantsu by bringing a person up onto his knees. People with knee or ankle problems might not be comfortable in the turtle position. Some might feel too vulnerable or awkward in it. But for those who are comfortable in it, it is a very powerful position for opening up both the neck and the back. Do not try to use this position with people too heavy for you to lift up into it. And do not leave a person too long in it.

If you think the turtle position would be appropriate, before beginning the session get into turtle yourself and, telling him you might be using this position sometime during the session to work on his back, ask the person if he is comfortable in this position.

Normally this position is used as a transition between your Tantsu work on the two sides. After finishing the work on the first side (the gall bladder meridian down the left leg), bring both his knees up as close as possible to his chest (he is still on his side). Position both his elbows bent in front of him.

1. **Raising the Turtle**. Up on your knees, straddle his lower legs. Reach over him and hook both your hands under his right hip. Slowly, without straining yourself, pull him up far enough to sit him back on your lap (you are sitting back on your heels, your legs spread). His sacrum is against your hara. Reach up and lifting one shoulder at a time, place his elbows directly under them so that his neck hangs freely, the weight of his head stretching it open.

2. **The Neck.** If easily accessible, you can reach under his shoulders and work his neck with the fingers of both hands. Don't pull his neck towards his chest, but lean into it with your fingers opening even more the spaces between the vertebras.

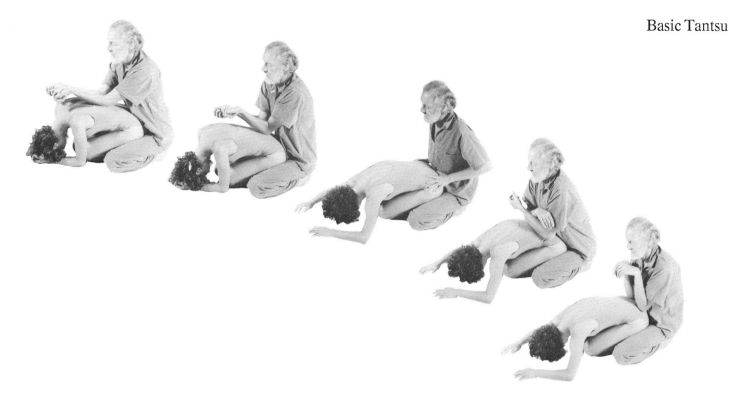

3. **The Neck Squeeze.** Take your arms out from under his arms. Hook your left fingers into his left shoulder and squeeze and work his neck with your right hand.

4. **The Shoulder Rock.** Hook the fingers of both hands into the tops of his shoulders and, keeping your arms straight, slowly rock back with your body. When you finish the rock tell him he can change his arms into whatever position is most comfortable for them.

5. **The Upper Back.** With your fingers still 'hooked', start working them down the first bladder meridian in the back (since you do not have the leverage to work deeply in this area, do not linger here until you get within range of your elbows).

6. **The Lower Back.** Switch to leaning in with both elbows (one on each side of the spine). Work down to just above the sacrum.

7. **The Sacrum.** Work down the points in the foramen in the sacrum and to each side of the tailbone with your thumbs.

8. **The Pump.** Place your forearms on his back as high up as you can comfortably reach, and a couple inches out from the first bladder meridian. As he breathes out 'pump' into your own hara. Move your forearms an inch or two down and continue pumping on down onto the buttocks.

9. **The Buttocks.** Lean into his buttocks with your elbows.

Make sure his arms won't get pinned under his legs, and that your left leg wont get pinned under his hip (move it out away from him). Roll him onto his left side and, moving behind his back, your foot level with his shoulder, do the Tantsu on his second side. (If your space is limited you can do a double roll, rolling him back on to his right side and continue rolling him onto his left side.)

This is a position you will not be able to use with everybody. For some it would be too intimate...and others would be too heavy for you to hold in this position. But for those with whom you can use it, it can be the most powerful of all the positions. It is the first position of Tantsu I developed, but because of its power I always include it at the end of a complete Tantsu session. Once someone is held in this position with its hara to first chakra connection, being held in any other position may feel anticlamatic and leave a person feeling abandoned.

I use the Lap position when I am doing a complete Tantsu. You can start the session with the Leg Cradle. After finishing the second leg, bring both knees back to the chest and roll the person to the right to do his first Side. Do the Turtle and the second Side. Bring both knees up and move into Lap. Follow the Lap with the Crossed Arm Pull and the Basic Co-Centering neck and head finish.

During the following you will be sitting under the person with your legs side straddle. Have a small rolled up towel nearby to place in front of your calf to take the person's weight if you feel he would be too heavy (or his spine too bony).

He is lying on his back. .

1. **Leg Rotation.** Press both his knees towards his chest and, kneeling, push behind his calves, raising him high enough to slip your left calf under his lower back. Hold both his ankles with your right hand and support yourself with your left hand on the floor as you slip side straddle under him, your right leg bent out to your right. Lower his left leg out over your right thigh and clasp his right leg to your chest (his thigh well above the knee in the crook of your left elbow and his foot in the crook of your right elbow, your fingers interlocked if possible). Holding his leg like a baby rotate it in both directions leaning back to stretch it and open the hip. (As you are doing this you can shift your leg under him into its most comfortable position. If it is still uncomfortable, you can place a rolled up towel in front of your leg.)

2. **The Leg Push.** Come out of your last rotation pushing his right calf towards his head with your left hand as you lean back with your right forearm onto his left leg. Hold.

3. **The Leg Pull.** Bend down and catch the back of his right knee over your left shoulder. Clasping his leg very close to you, making sure his knee does not slip off your shoulder, lean back to stretch.

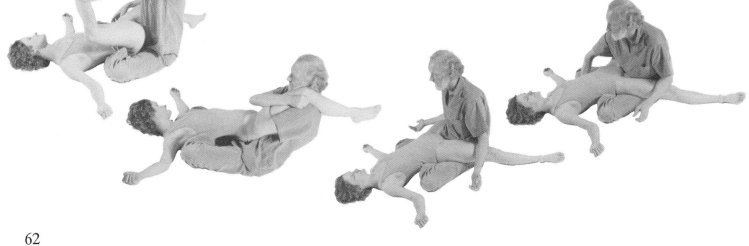

If your legs are not comfortable in their side straddle position under him, you can introduce a move at this point to straighten and reverse them. You can lean his legs forward and stand, pulling up his legs to swing his back as in the Expanded Co-centering; and then return with your right calf under him and your left leg out to the side, to continue the work with the second leg.

4. **The Left Leg.** Lay his right leg to your left side and hold his left leg to your chest (his foot in the crook of your left elbow, etc.) and rotate, pull and push as above.

5. **The Lean back.** Lay his left leg to your right side. Lean back on both legs with your forearms in three places working towards his knees.

6. **The Back Lift.** Hold down his right leg with your left forearm (arching his back up) and slip your right fist under the left side of his back (as high up as you can comfortably reach). Slip your left fist under the right side (your knuckles should be parallel to the spine under the first bladder meridians). As he breathes out lift gently with both fists (eliminate the lifting with people with back problems that might be worsened with arching). Continue lifting with each outbreath, working down to the lower back. Hold.

7. **The Hara.** Keep your right fist raising the lower back as you slip out your left hand and lay it across the hara just below the navel. Hold. Slip out your right hand and work the complete hara pattern, leaning in with your own hara on each outbreath.

8. **Out from Under.** Hold the hara with your left hand and the heart chakra with your right hand. Lift off both hands and, placing his feet against your chest, lean into his feet with your chest to slip out. Stand and, straightening them, lower his legs. Squatting back, pull both his feet by the ankles. Holding the tops of his feet near the toes, press them down.

The following expansion incorporates both work on the upper back from above the head and additional work on the legs and feet. They are presented together here for convenience. Normally, depending on the person's needs, expand the face down in only one of these directions, and then, only with people you are certain can stay comfortable in this position.

1. **The Basic Rock.** Facing his back, rock as in Basic.

2. **The Catwalk.** When your left hand has 'walked' up to the upper back, leave it there as you move into a position above his head. Sit seiza placing the heels of your hands between his upper spine and the upper corner of his shoulder blades (fingers outward). Start slowly rocking alternate hands into his upper back like a cat kneeding (the direction of your rock towards his hips, not towards the floor).

3. **The Upper Back.** Keep your middle finger hooked into Bladder 10 under the occiput (on the side he is facing) and lean with your elbow into Bladder 11 (the side he is facing). Hold. Lean into the next four or five Bladder points down the upper back.

4. **The Pump Down.** Still holding the occiput with your left hand, place your forearm just past where your elbow stopped (without touching the spine). As he breathes out 'pump' your forearm towards his sacrum (not towards the floor). Continue with faster pumping until you reach the edge of the sacrum. Continue holding the occiput firmly as you lean into the sacrum, stretching the spine.

5. **The Head Turn.** Hold the top of his head with one hand and squeeze down the back of his neck with the other. Gently lift and turn his head to the other side. Repeat the squeeze down the neck, hook your middle finger under his occiput and repeat the above down this side of the back

6. **The Crossed Arm Return.** Cross your arms (your right on top) and lean the heels of your hands into the underside of his scapulas as he breathes out. As he breathes in move back to his left side, your raised left knee straddling his arm, your right knee on the floor. As he breathes out lean into his upper back with both hands (fingers outward). As he breathes in move down a little farther. Lean in on the next outbreath. Continue, stopping before you drop below the rib cage. Lower your knee to the floor. Place the heels of both hands to the right side of his spine and lean into three places as in Basic.

7. **The Double Mother.** Lean into Bladder 36 at the top of his right leg with your right knee.

Continue mothering with both the heel of your left hand (still behind the heart center) and your knee as you work gently down the Bladder meridian (the far side of his spine) with your right elbow, your arm kept open.

8. **The Near Side.** Slip the heel of your left hand to the near side of his spine (between spine and scapula). Lean your right knee into the side of his left buttock. Place your right hand just below your left hand and work down this side of the spine, first with the heel of your hand and then with your elbow.

9. **The Sacrum.** With your feet between his calves, place your knees in the very tops of his legs (without putting pressure on his knees) and with both thumbs lean into the points down the sacrum and to the sides of the tailbone (If this is not comfortable, work down the sacrum as in the Expanded Co-centering). Move back to his left side and stretch his spine with crossed arms and work down the buttock and the back of his thigh as in the Expanded Co-centering.

10. **The Knee Hold.** Slip your right hand under his left knee and move down laying his left foot across your right thigh (you are sitting seiza facing his knee). Hold his left knee from underneath with your right hand. Lay your left forearm across the back of his knee and gently work the knee from underneath with your right hand. Work lightly down the midline of his calf with your left elbow (Bladder meridian).

11. **The Foot Bend.** Without letting go of his knee (if possible), pick up his foot with your left hand, swinging it up until just the part near his toes is still under your armpit. Lean into his foot stretching it while holding firmly his heel with your left thumb and forefinger in Bladder 62 and Kidney 6.

12. **The Foot Push.** Hold his leg behind the ankle with your right hand while your left hand pushes his foot forward (both your arms are straight).

13. **Optional Footwork.** Pincer holding Bladder 62 and Kidney 6 with your left hand, lower his foot across the top of your left thigh (you are sitting seiza facing his opposite foot). Lean into three places down the bottom of his foot with your right forearm. Lean into four or five places in a clockwise circle with your elbow, starting from and returning to Kidney 1.

14. **The Second Leg**. Move to his right side. Lean into his sacrum with your right hand while your left hand presses his left foot (still in your hand) towards his left buttock. Work as above down his right leg and foot. Roll him over as in Basic.

The Side Position

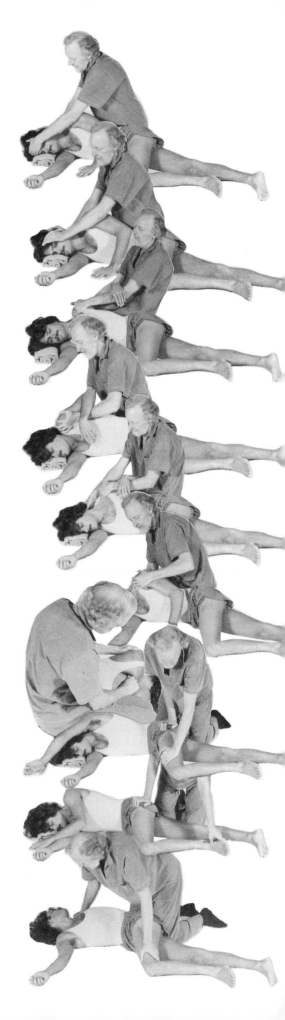

This form can follow the Face Down Co-centering. Roll him onto his right side from the face down position, his lower leg straight and the leg you pulled to roll him (his left) bent in front of him. Pull his right arm out in front of him. Make sure his back is straight and on a plane perpendicular to the floor. Place a rolled up towel under his head and sit seiza alongside his back (the side of your hip against his lower back).

1. **The Jaw.** Simultaneously place your left hand over his forehead, and the heel of your right hand under his occiput. Lean in with your right hand gradually increasing the pressure. Hold. Keeping the fingers of your left hand touching his forehead (without pressing his eyes), gently lean the heel of your left hand into the jaw hinge area. Hold.

2. **The Shoulder Pull.** Remove your left hand and, slipping it under his wrist to pick up his left arm, hook your hand around his shoulder. Remove your right hand and place it over your left hand. Lean back pulling his shoulder until his head is lifted off the towel. Hold.

3. **The Shoulder Rotation.** Lean forward and rotate his shoulder, clasping it between the heels of your hands, stretching it to all sides. Rotate both directions. Come out of the last rotation leaning back.

4. **The Neck Stretch.** Lean back, pulling his shoulder, until his head lifts off the towel. Hold. Maintaining the stretch of his neck with your left hand, reach out with your right thumb and, starting just under the occipital ridge, hold one breath each three places down the line being stretched: Gall Bladder 20, the back of his neck, and Gall Bladder 21 in the top of his shoulder. Hold.

5. **The Shoulder Blade.** Slip your right thumb under the upper corner of his left scapula. Slip your left hand out from under his left arm and hold his upper left arm from above. As he breathes out lean down on his upper left arm sliding the scapula over your right thumb. Slide the scapula up as he breathes in and replant right thumb down an inch or two further down the scapula. Lean in with your left hand on the next outbreath. Continue the rest of the way down the scapula.

6. **The Rib Cage.** Up on both knees facing his head, clasp his ribcage and work down to his waist leaning gently without pressure, a rib between the thumbs of your splayed hands each time.

7. **Gall Bladder.** Both arms straight, lean the heel of your right hand into Gall Bladder 30 in his hip joint while the heel of your left hand works down the midline of his leg. Hold Gall Bladder 40(just below his ankle) with your left thumb (your right hand still on 30.) Hold..

8. **The Roll Over.** With your right hand pick up his left arm and lay it out behind his back. Gently push his shoulder back to twist stretch his spine. Straighten his left leg. Bend his right leg and pull it across his left leg rolling him onto his left side. Repeat the above. Roll him onto his back and do the face up work.

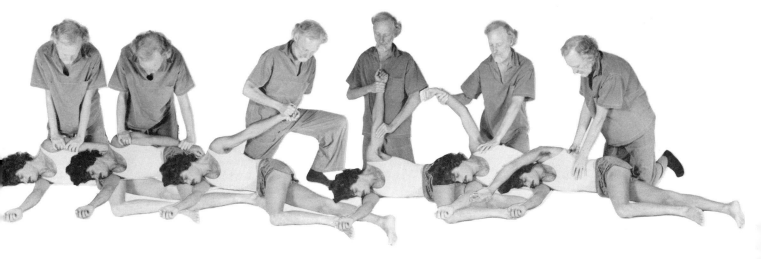

Expansions to this form that incorporate work on the arms. All or part of the following can be incorporated into this pattern just after the work under the shoulder blade(5).

5a. The Arm Back. Bring his left arm behind his back onto your lap and work individual points.

5b.. Leaning down the Arm. Lay his left arm (straightened) on his side and, getting up on both knees facing his back, grasp with both hands and lean into his upper arm (his back staying on a plane perpindicular to the floor). Mother, grasping the top of his arm with your right hand, as your left hand, on each outbreath grasps and leans into a place further down the arm until it arrives at the wrist.

5c. **The Arm Pull.** Lift your left knee and pivot on your right knee to face his feet as, with both hands you pick up his hand and pull his arm. The fingers of both hands should be in his palm pulling open his hand. (At this point you can add pulls of the individual fingers, either with both hands simultaneously, each pulling a finger, or with one hand holding the wrist while the other pulls).

5d. **The Arm Raise.** Holding his wrist to maintain a pull, swing his arm up vertical at the same time as you drop your left knee back down to the floor and turn to face his arm. Hold his arm to your chest. Clasp his upper arm with the fingers and thumb of your left hand and, still holding his wrist with your right hand, squeeze and rock up and back as he breathes out. Continue working this way to the wrist.

5e. **The Arm Rotation.** Drop your left hand to lay across his armpit and, holding his forearm just below the elbow, rotate his arm in a clockwise direction.

5f. **The Heart Stretch.** Lay his arm up over his head. Mother Heart 7 in his wrist with your right thumb while your left hand (the part just below your fingers) works gently out the Heart meridian. Clasp his rib cage and continue as in 6 above.

The Sitting Position

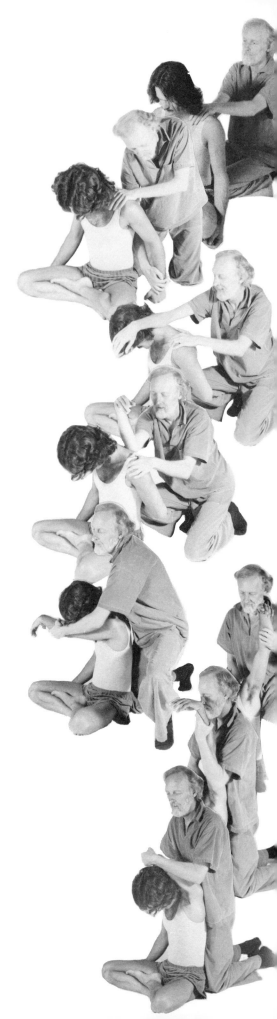

The sitting position is useful when your time, or the space available, is limited. It can also be used as the first position of a complete session. In Japan it is usually done with someone sitting seiza, but in this country fewer people are used to sitting in that position. When you work on someone sitting on the floor crosslegged it is necessary to constantly be providing support to his back. In the sequence below that support is provided by your knees. If you have trouble using your knees, or they do not seem appropriate for the person you are working with, try other ways of supporting the back. One way that will work with most people is to make an A frame of your legs, your right knee at the base of his spine, and your other out to the side so that you can lean his spine back against your right leg (making certain his head is comfortable on the side of your chest). This position, a variant to the one below, gives you access to the chest, shoulders, neck and head on which you can work freestyle.

Have your partner sit on the floor, legs comfortably crossed. Ask him if he has any problems with his back or anything you should know. Tell him to let you know if anything is uncomfortable.

1. **Straightening the back.** Sit 'seiza' behind him, your knees a couple inches from him, and center yourself. Simultaneously place your left hand on his left shoulder and your right hand over the spine between his scapulas. Hold, connecting to his breathing. Slide your right hand down his spine, straightening his back as needed. Hold his lower back.

2. **The Forearm down the Neck.** Without taking your left hand off his shoulder, reach down with your right hand and bring his left arm behind his back. See if it can be raised bent comfortably as high as his lowest ribs. If it can't, lower it to the floor behind him. If it can, hold it raised. Shift your body so that you are towards his right side at about a 45 degree angle to his back, place your right knee just to the right of his spine between his rib cage and sacrum. Lower his left hand (palm up) on your knee. Maintain constant support with your knee. Make sure it is comfortable and not pressing into his kidney. Gently lean the soft side of your right forearm into his occiput, the middle of his neck, and the base of his neck, each time pulling his shoulder down. Continue leaning in around the shoulder blade each time pulling his shoulder back.

3. **The Shoulder Blade.** Still holding his shoulder with your left hand, place your right elbow between his scapula and neck. Say 'Take a deep breath and let it all the way out...' As he breathes out lean in with your elbow while pulling his shoulder back. On the inbreath let his shoulder return forward and slide your elbow down an inch or two. On the next out breath again lean in under his scapula and pull his shoulder back. Repeat a couple more times.

4. **The Arm Rotation.** Place the Karate side of your right hand firmly behind his upper left scapula. Remove your left hand from his shoulder and hold his left arm just below the elbow. Dropping your right knee to the floor at the base of his spine, bring his left arm around in front of him. Raise your left knee. Dancing your raised knee forward as his arm comes to his front, rotate his arm in wide circles (in the direction up towards his nose).

5. **The Lung Stretch.** Come out of the rotation stretching his arm back at an angle 45 degrees up from horizontal (the Lung meridian stretch). Maintain firm support with your Karate hand, still between his neck and shoulder blade, bracing it against the side of your body.

6. **The Circulation Stretch.** Lower his arm, dropping your left knee to the floor. Swing his arm up and stretch it back linking your arm around it. (Circulation meridian stretch). Maintain firm support.

7. **Heart Stretch.** Lower his arm and swing it up behind his head while moving (nudging his head forward on the way) your right hand onto his right shoulder to keep him upright. Holding his elbow loosely lean your left forearm against his lower arm gently stretching it towards his right shoulder (heart meridian stretch).

8. **The Second Arm.** Lower his left arm and, keeping your right hand on his right shoulder, with your left hand draw his right arm behind his back. Repeat 2-7 on the right side.

9. **The Lift Off.** Both hands on his shoulders, stand and place the outside of your right leg against his spine. With both thumbs work out the tops of his shoulders and, with both hands, squeeze down his upper arms. Just before his elbows swing his arms up, letting them slide through your hands. Hold them just below the wrists to your side. Bend at the waist and lift your right heel to stretch his whole body.

10. **The Butterfly.** Lower and, keeping his upper arms parallel to the floor, draw his arms back (butterfly wings), opening his chest. Still holding the wrists, raise his arms slightly, swing them forward and draw them back again. Repeat several times. Hold them even more open the last time(your leg still bracing his spine).

11. **The Twist.** Lower his arms. Place your left hand in front of his left shoulder and your right hand behind his right shoulder. Place your right knee behind your right hand and, keeping his spine straight, twist him to the left. Reverse the positioning of your hands and knees and twist him to the right. If you are going on to the face down position, roll him onto the floor. Straighten his body, pulling first his legs, and then his arms, laying them out to the sides.

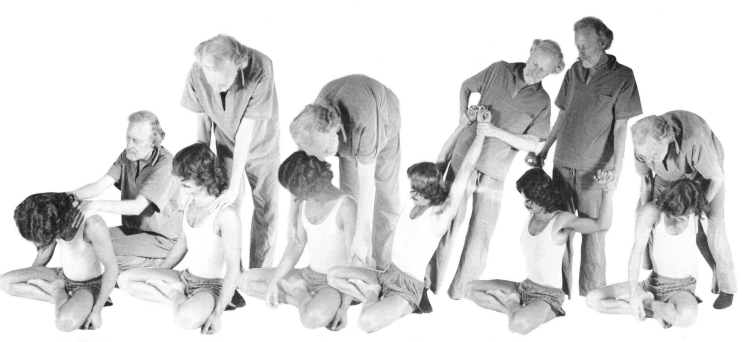

Start behind his back as in Basic, your toes level with the top of his shoulder.

1. **Heart and Mind.** Simultaneously pick up his left forearm with your left hand and his head with your right hand. While pulling his left arm and lifting his head, slide your right thigh under his head right up against his shoulders. Lay his left arm comfortably across your left leg and his neck over your right. Place your left hand on his heart chakra and, making sure his neck is completely supported by your leg and his head is not turned to either side, place your right hand across his forehead centered on his third eye. Hold feeling the connection between these two chakras (your own back should be as straight as is comfortable).

2. **Lung Area.** Still holding his forehead, lean across the upper corner of his chest (an area related to the lung meridian) with your left forearm. Hold.

3. **Jaw.** Keeping your forearm in contact with the Lung area, hold and pull down his chin with your left hand opening his mouth. Say 'let your jaw drop'. When his mouth opens lean gently into the jaw hinge area with the heel of your left hand. Hold.

4. **Points around the Eye.** Still holding his forehead with your right hand, lightly place the middle finger of your left hand in Bladder 2 under the inside corner of his eyebrow. With the same finger work points in a circle around the eye: Large Intestine 20, Stomach 3, Small Intestine 18, and Gall Bladder l.

5. **Crown.** Slide your left hand onto the forehead replacing your right hand as it moves up and, with four fingers pressing in, works along the top of the head. Hold the crown chakra as in the Basic Side. Continue as in Basic, crossing under with your right hand to hold the Heart chakra and squeezing out the arm. Hold the Circulation point in the hand.

6. **The Lung Meridian.** Leaning your forearm across lung 1, hold lung 6 with your right thumb while your left thumb holds lung 9 in his wrist.

7. **The Large Intestine Meridian**. Still leaning into Lung 1, bend his wrist forward and hold Large Intestine 4 with your left thumb while your right thumb holds 11 in the elbow. Hold. Bend and rotate his wrist. Stretch and rotate his arm as in the Basic Side.

8. **The Heart Meridian.** Lay his arm up over his head and mother Heart 1 in the armpit with your left palm while the fingers of your right hand press out his Heart meridian to the wrist.

9. **The Rib Cage.** Lay your right forearm (hand towards you) across his armpit while your left forearm (hand away) gently works down his rib cage. Clasp his waist with your forearms. Pull his leg, rest, and move into the position above his head as in Basic.

Do all the Basic moves in the second position. If you are not planning to use the Turtle, before going to the third position, return to the first position behind his back and insert the following.

10. **The Back Rock**. Place your hands side by side on his upper back, their heels about an inch above his spine. Gently rock him. Keep your right hand rocking where it is and slowly 'walk' your rocking left hand down to his sacrum.

11. **The Bladder Meridian.** Place your right thumb in the heart area of the Bladder meridian to mother with, while you work all the way down the meridian to the side of the tailbone with your left thumb, leaning in with each outbreath. Hook your left fingers around his tail bone as your right thumb and forefinger leans into the Bladder 10 points under the occiput. Hold.

Move down to below his hips.

12. **The Arm Pull.** As you move into the third position (below his hips) take his arm. Sit on your heels, your knees clasping him, and pull his wrist with your left hand while your right pushes (towards his shoulder) and squeezes, working all the way down his arm.

13. **The Finger Pull.** Hold his wrist with your right hand while your left hand pulls his thumb and fingers. Lay his wrist over your arm and rotate his shoulder as in Basic.

14. **Forearm down the Back.** When you come out of the last rotation pull his arm forward while working around his shoulder and down his back with your right forearm. Hold his lower back with your right forearm and his thigh with your left forearm. Squeeze and hold. Rotate his hip, continue and finish as in the Basic Side.

It is not necessary to duplicate every move on both sides. Feel free to innovate. Try doing everything on the second side from one or two positions. If I use the Turtle, I often do the whole second side from the position below the hips, which maintains support of the first chakra (which will be continued into the Lap position).

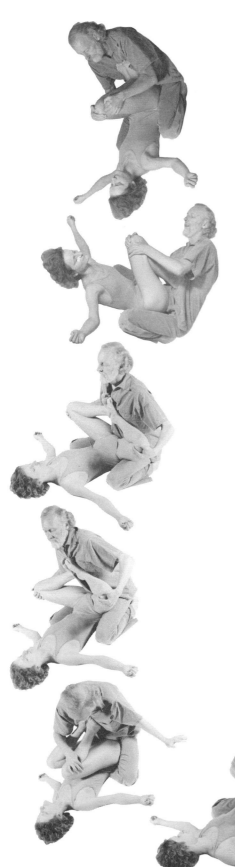

The following introduces a prologue to the Basic Lap work and incorporates more detailed pointwork on the legs in this position. Have a rolled up towel handy to protect your calf when it is slipped under the back.

He is lying on his back.

1. **Hara-Sacrum.** Press both his knees towards his chest and, kneeling, push behind his calves. Pressing his legs up beside his head (being careful not to stretch his neck too far forward), move closer to him until your hara is against his sacrum with your knees spread a little, sit back on your heels, your hara still against his sacrum.

2. **Hip Rotation.** Press his feet against your chest and, holding his knees with both hands, rotate his hips in both directions.

3. **Spread Leg Rotation.** Spread his knees and, with his feet against your chest (or crossed and tucked under your arms if he is tall), rotate his hips in both directions.

4. **Spread Leg Rock.** Holding his feet pressed against each other on your chest, keep his knees pulled apart as your chest rocks into his feet.

5. **Leg Rotation.** Place your left hand on the floor and lean into his knees (bent up) with your right forearm as you switch your legs into side straddle, your left lower leg under his lower back and your right leg bent out to your side. Lower his left leg out to your side over your right leg and clasp his right leg to your chest (his thigh in the crook of your left elbow and his foot in the crook of your right elbow, your fingers interlocked if possible). Holding his leg like a baby rotate it in both directions leaning back to stretch it and open the hip. (As you are doing this you can shift your leg under him into its most comfortable position. If it is still uncomfortable, you can place a rolled up towel in front of your leg.)

6. **Stomach Meridian.** Come out of the rotation leaning into Stomach 36 with your left thumb (pressing his knee towards his shoulder and the side of your body holding his foot turned inward). Work the next three points down the stomach meridian with your right thumb.

7. **The Kidney Meridian.** Lean his still bent leg towards the opposite shoulder with your right hand while your left elbow works the kidney meridian down the thigh from the knee (where Masunaga locates it, just to the outside of the Bladder meridian).

8. **The Bladder Meridian.** Slip your left elbow into bladder 36 at the top of his leg, and pincer hold Kidney 6 and Bladder 62 below his ankle with your left thumb and forefinger, while your right thumb holds across the back of his knee. Hold. Work up the midline of his calf with your right thumb. Hold his knee with your right hand while your left elbow works up the midline of his thigh.

9. **The Leg Push.** As in the Basic Lap, push his right calf towards his head with your left hand as you lean back with your right forearm on his left leg.

10. **The Leg Pull.** As in the Basic Lap bend down and catch the back of his right knee over your left shoulder. Holding his leg to you lean back to stretch.

11. **The Crossover Stretch.** Push his right leg forward again, while, this time, pulling his left arm by the wrist. Hold. If it doesn't look like the back of his elbow can wrap around the back of his knee, lower both arm and leg and proceed to move 12 below. If it does look like it can, then pull his arm around the back of his knee. Still holding his wrist, slip around (to the inside of) his right foot and pull his left shoulder with your left hand. Let go of his left wrist and, with your right hand, work around the back of his shoulder, and down his back. Let go of his shoulder and lay his left arm back out to his side.

12. **The Second Leg.** Lay his right leg to your left side and do a mirror image of the above with his left leg.

13. **The Finish.** Lay his left leg to your right side. Lean back on both legs with your forearms working towards his knees, and continue with the work under the back, and in the hara; and finish as in the Basic Lap.

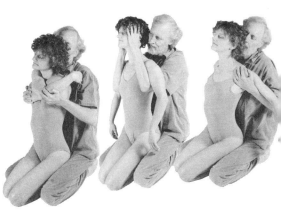

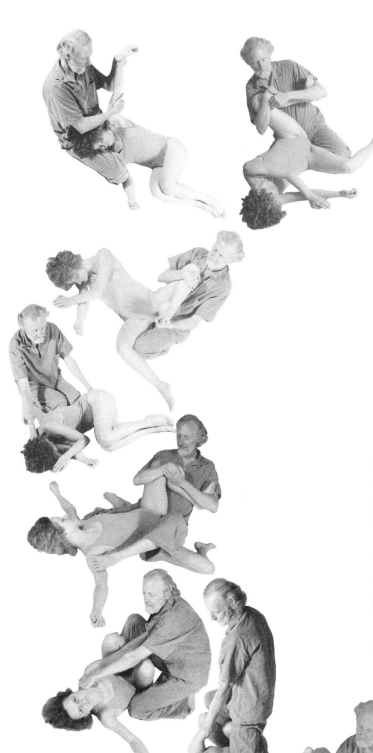

Freestyle is the adapting and combining of the forms in this book to individualize each session according to the needs of your shiatsu partner. it is answering the calls of those places that suddenly cry for attention. Trust your impulse. The particular order of the sequences in this book are not sacrosanct. They are meant to be a framework that insures the body as a whole and all its meridian-pairs will receive some attention during a session. Within that framework feel free to explore and create. The more people you work with the more you will come to realize that each one is different. The more you learn to do the sequences in this book without having to think about what comes next, the more you can be with each person in the moment. The more you are with a person, connected with your whole being, the more your 'being' will know just what that person needs. This is the basis of intuition (and the basis of a 'good touch'). Trust your intuition and it will grow. Go where you feel called. Stay until you feel completion within yourself. Introduce movement, or rocking or vibration when you feel it coming out of your own being. Leave the sequence and return to it. Or go on to another. But always keep an eye on your partner. Be aware of the effects of what you are doing. Stay within his limits. Be with him.

Free Form is following no sequence. It is spontaneously moving with someone to the rhythms of the energy being released. When it happens you feel your connection to your partner on a completely different and more creative plane or dimension. It may begin as a feeling of movement rising in your own body, carrying both you and your partner along, as you find yourselves flowing from one position to another, cradling and rocking and stretching and holding in ways you never have before. (And when it does happen, don't feel required to keep working in this mode throughout the session. Feel free to return to the sequences anytime.) You may find this more likely to happen when you are working with someone smaller, particularly if they are someone, such as a dancer, to whom movement is a natural way of being. It is more difficult with someone larger, but not impossible as I was shown one time by the woman who organizes my classes in Munich, who, after I had just demonstrated Free Form, was paired with someone twice her size. She looked at him and saw how she could never get into the positions I had just moved through. The utter impossibility of it was a koan that emptied her mind. She saw herself making a giant snowman, and rolled over and over him rolling up the snow. He loved it.

75

MERIDIAN PAIR STRETCHES

Lung/Large Intestine. To stretch the meridians of the outside, stand, feet apart, knees not locked. Center. Link your thumbs behind your back. As you breathe out raise your arms up behind you and, keeping your legs straight, drop your torso forward. Settle into it a little deeper on each outbreath. Hold. Slowly come up.

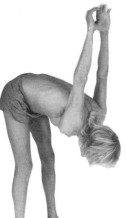

The following stretches can help you open your own meridians. There is a stretch for each meridian pair. Begin with centering (letting everything settle into your center as you breathe out). Keep centered throughout. Settle into the stretches on an outbreath. Hold the stretch as you breathe in being aware of any tension you feel along the meridians. Enjoy the letting go, the opening up of the meridians as you settle a little deeper into the stretch on each subsequent outbreath. Do not bounce or force yourself to stay in any position that is uncomfortable.

Heart/Small Intestine. To stretch the meridians of the inside, sit with your feet against each other and pulled into you as close as possible. Your knees should be as low as possible. Hold your feet with both hands and roll forward. Feel how you are stretching into your inside.

Stomach/Spleen. To stretch the meridians of the front you bend back. (Omit this stretch if you have any problem with your lower back or knees which might be aggravated by back bends.) Sit seiza between your heels. If you can do it without straining your lower back or your knees, lay back flat on the floor and, if comfortable, straighten your arms out on the floor up over your head. To avoid straining your back, roll to the side to come up.

Bladder/Kidney. To stretch the meridians of the back, sit on the floor with your legs straightened out in front of you. Raise your arms up in the air, and, as you breathe out, swing forward, keeping your knees straight.

Circulation/Triple Heater. To stretch the meridian of the surface. If you are used to lotus, sit lotus. If not, sit half lotus or cross-legged. Crossing your arms, hold your knees with both hands and roll forward as you breathe out.

Gall Bladder/Liver. To stretch the meridians of the sides, spread your legs as wide out to the sides as possible (keeping them straight). Clasp your hands high over your head (palms upward) and stretch to one side...And then to the other. Finish with a stretch forward between your spread legs (to stretch the central meridians). Follow this with one of the meditations of the next section.

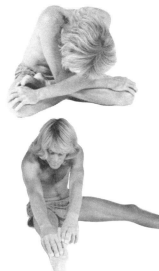

AN ANATOMY OF ENERGY

My training in Zen Shiatsu taught me to work from the hara, to move from it and, as I lean into a place on someone's body, to feel the release in my own hara (a process I call earlier in this book 'center holding'). Working in water I find that when I float and move someone level with my chest I feel I am moving them with my heart center. I feel a resonating in that chakra as it becomes more open. When I finish against the wall with the person straddling my leg and lift my hand off their third eye, I often feel our two energies rise up our backs and, sometimes, intertwining, rising still higher up into an incredible brightness.

There are at least three different states of energy involved: circulating, resonating, and rising. The energy in the meridians is circulating through our bodies. The energy in our chakras is resonating. And the energy up the back is rising.

As I developed Co-centering I came to realize how much power there is in repeatedly connecting and reconnecting our three basic centers. Our body center in the hara is the center of the energy circulating through our meridians which maintains our physical life; our heart center, the center of our chakras' resonating energy with which we connect to others; and the mind center, the center through which our energy rises to connect us to higher realities.

I had been thinking for some time about the nature of these three centers and their relationship to the other chakras and the meridians when I came across a statement by Lao Tzu which made it immediately clear: *The Tao gives birth to the One. The One gives birth to the Two. The Two to the Three. And the Three to the Ten Thousand.* Creation itself is continuously repeated in the inter-relationships between chakras, meridians and the movements of energy in each of us.

To make this clear to my students I developed a sequence of meditations through which they could get in touch with these inter-relationships by experiencing them in their own bodies (the only way you can really 'know' any form of energy). These meditations supplement and bring into perspective what students feel in their own bodies as they learn and practice Bodywork Tantra. The meditations combine with the bodywork to create a powerful process for self realization.

In the following the meditations are italicized. After each there are discussions about the chakras encountered and their related meridians. All the chakras and meridians are covered and the points encountered in this book are located. (A body inch is a distance proportionate to each person. To find this measurement on yourself you can make a ruler based on the 12 body inches there are between the creases of your elbow and your wrist on the inside of your arm. A rule of thumb is that the breadth of the first joint of your thumb is one body inch.)

Before starting each meditation do the stretches of the last section to get the energy flowing. Then, except for the one where you are told to stand, sit in a position which helps you keep your back straight. If you can not sit comfortably in lotus or seiza, you can sit on the edge of a chair. In all of these you will be using the natural rhythm of breathing as a vehicle to connect you to the most basic movements of energy in your body. Our breathing alternates between an active (yang) and a passive (yin) phase. On the inbreath our muscles lower the diaphragm and expand the chest. On the exhalation they relax and the subsequent collapse forces the air out. The more relaxed you become the deeper and slower the breathing becomes. A cassette of these meditations is available from the school.

Sit comfortably, your back straight. Let your shoulders and neck relax. Be aware of your hara (abdomen). As you breathe out feel a settling into your hara. As you breathe in feel a rising up your back. And a settling back into your hara as you breathe out. Feel the rising up your back as you breathe in as a wave spreading out to all parts of your body. And, as you breathe out, feel how all those parts let go, and settling, empty into the hara. Be aware of any part that doesn't let go as much as the rest. That is where you are carrying tension (blocked energy). The next time you breathe in fill that part even more. And let it empty as you breathe out...Let everything settle and empty into your hara everytime you breathe out...and rise up your back everytime you breathe in.

Be aware of what happens at the bottom of the breath when everything empties into the hara. It is a bowl at the base of the spine - the navel the front, the sacrum the back, and the perineum, between your legs, the bottom. Feel how at the very bottom of the breath, for a moment, the bowl itself is empty. Feel that emptiness in the bottom of that bowl, in the first chakra. It is here where our energy empties back into the void, a state in which it is pure potential. The more completely you let yourself go and empty into that void, the more powerful the rise you will feel up your back as you breathe in.

The Tao

I had been using the above meditation for some time when I read Lao Tzu's statement and realized that what I had felt in the void in the first chakra is the Tao, the 'undifferentiated', the 'mother of all beings'. In tantra the first chakra is called the powerhouse of all the other chakras. The Chinese term for the perineum means the collection point of all yin energy. It is also known as the Gate of Death and Life.

In tantric and taoist sexual practices incredible energy can be directed upward from this chakra repeatedly and without limit. But only if there is first a complete letting go into it, a not trying.

In both Watsu and Tantsu I find that if I hold people in such a way their first chakra is supported on my leg or on my lap while I work the rest of their body, there is a greater sense of connection; they experience a deeper calm and let go more.

Its location in the perineum is midway between where we 'let go' of liquid and solid waste, where we literally 'void' ourselves. It is an area that we guard closely. Much fear and 'holding' has been built up in this area through excessive toilet training and/or sexual violence (including the violence of labeling this area and its associated functions 'dirty'). Consequently there is much to let go of when we find we can be held in this area in a completely non-judgemental, non-threatening way. The nature of the first chakra becomes even clearer when we look at the meridian pair related to it, the Bladder/Kidney.

Bladder

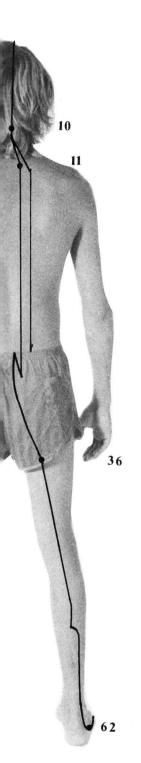

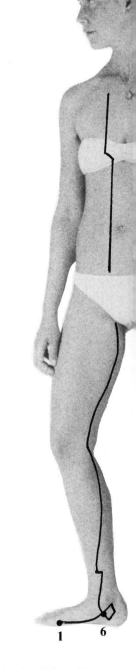

The Bladder meridian begins to the inside of the eyes. It runs up over the top of the head and all the way down the back. It is connected to the Kidney meridian which begins in the bottom of the foot and ends in the chest just below the clavicle.

The primary function of this meridian pair is purification through elimination. It governs all eliminatory processes. Traditionally each pair is associated with an element, a color, a period of life, an emotional state, etc. This pair is associated with water, the color black, death, and fear. Death is the ultimate purification through elimination. These are the meridians of the back, what we leave behind us, or, if unable to leave, carry on our back.

A back pain is usually something we are holding onto, not letting go (not 'eliminating'). An inability to let go of tension in other meridians eventually shows up as a tightness or weakness in a particular area of the back (see chart on page 29). The area where held tension in the Bladder meridian itself shows up is the bottom of the spine, the sacrum. The sacrum is also associated with the first chakra. It is the area where rising energy begins its ascent up through the spine. Our not letting go weakens this ascent both by denying the first chakra the energy to purify and recycle, and by turning up as tension in the back where it constricts whatever is rising.

When it is the Bladder/Kidney itself that is not letting go that ascent is constricted from the beginning (the sacrum), and further weakened by the fact the meridians responsible for assisting the other meridians to let go are themselves bound up. This situation, and its accompanying growing fear of letting go, can only worsen if left to itself.

Work on the back and the sacrum, and helping people 'let go' in this area increases the effectiveness of work on any other part the body. The first chakra is the first chakra. And to the degree it is closed down and we are not in touch with the Tao in ourselves, we will not be able to be in touch with the other states of energy.

Kidney 1. Midway across the ball of the foot almost one third the distance from the tip of the middle toe to the heel. **6.** Depression immediately below the ankle.

Bladder 2. Depression at the inner corner of the eyebrow. **10.** Just below the top cervical vertebra. **11.** 1.5 body inches lateral to the lower border of the first thoracic vertebra's spinous process. **36.** Base of hip at thighbone. **62..** Depression below the tip of the external malleolus.

Begin, as in the previous meditation, with stretching, and then, sitting, your back straight. Feel everything settling, emptying into your hara as you breathe out...and rising up your back, a wave spreading to all parts of your body, as you breathe in. Feel how all those parts let go and settle and empty into the hara as you breathe out. Feel how, at the very bottom, the hara itself is empty. And how the more you let go into that emptiness at the bottom of the hara, the more rises up your back as you breathe in. Enjoy, savor the feeling of just completely letting yourself go into that void at the bottom of the breath. It is the Tao. Let yourself go into it a little deeper and stay a little longer at the bottom of each breath. Feel how, as the breath is about to start back up, that void surrounds the base of your spine like a dark bulb around the stalk of a lily. And as you breathe in feel how everything rises up that stalk, higher and higher. And how at the very top of your breath there is as much a fullness as there is an emptiness at the bottom. The Tao gives birth to the One. At the top of each breath rest a little longer in that fullness. There everything exists in its fullest, brightest state. Everything is light. Feel that light growing the longer you stay up at the top of the breath. It is a light that you have a place in, that you are one with, that everything is one with. And if anything is preventing you from feeling yourself one with it now, it is the effort you are putting into trying to rise up to it. There is no need. You are already one with it. And as you breathe out settling back into the void, let go of all effort, of all desire. Let it all empty back into the Tao. Let everything empty into the Tao, like the slow falling of snow growing darker and darker as it disappears below. And as you breathe in let yourself be taken all the way back up into, inside that light. Being inside light is entirely different from seeing light. It is a shining out to all sides.

The Crown

The crown chakra sits on top, just over the top, of our head. It is our godhead. It is where our energy enters into its fullest state, where it is (where we are) one with everything.

I one time experienced a vision in which I rose towards clouds of light, a city of light I couldn't quite rise up into, and when I realized I couldn't because I was trying too hard, and stopped trying, light poured down on me from those clouds in a gentle golden, loving rain.

And another time I saw that city above, and this time I called upon spirit guides for help and suddenly found myself inside that light. It is totally different from the streets and buildings of light I had seen from below. It is being light. It is shining out to all sides - long rays of light whirling worlds and universes.

The crown chakra is the place of our being in light. And all our various experiences of divine light, and of beings of light, come down and draw us back up into that place of absolute unity.

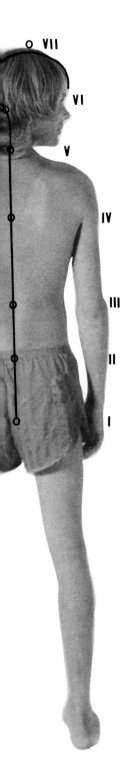

The meridian pair related to the crown chakra is the governing vessel and the conception vessel. These are the meridians of the midline. The governing vessel begins below the tail bone and rises up the middle of the spine up over the head. The conception vessel flows down the front to the perineum. The Taoists connect these two in a continuous cycle of energy which they call the microcosmic circuit.

In Acupuncture these meridians are called the lake of energy out of which the other meridians flow like rivers. Since the feeling of rising up the back has a very strong yang feeling, and the settling down the front, a yin, when I first read Lao Tze's statement I saw these as the Two that are born out of the One; a yin/yang polarization of the unity of the crown chakra; an archetype for the other chakras whose related meridian pairs are polarizations of the energy that exists in its unified state in the chakra. The polarized state is the state the energy must be in to fullfill its function in maintaining our physical life; the unified state, the state it must be in to connect with other chakras.

The rising up the back is creation, the birth of the One out of the Tao. And the settling down the front, the return into the Tao. This rising up the back in Kundalini is sometimes accompanied with extremely intense and/or disturbing experiences. This may happen when it is suddenly let out after being bottled up a long time. Or it may have to do with incomplete letting go and the resulting constricting tension in the back.

The relationship between the Tao and the One should make it clear that those who start a spiritual practice by cutting off their bodies are pursuing a very difficult course. The first chakra, and the functions related to that area, have been badly maligned. The ability to accept and let go into the Tao is a prerequisite to physical and spirital health.

At the other end of the spectrum are those who have cut their heads (and hearts) off from their bodies, and live for sexual conquest and power without an inkling of how much greater joy they could experience (and share with their partners) in a sexual practice which is based on letting go into the Tao and feeling the energy rise up the back (opening the heart on its way up).

The Chakras: I. In the perineum, between the legs midway between the genitals and the anus. **II.** Just below the navel. **III.** In the solar plexus. **IV.** Between the breasts. **V.** On the throat. **VI.** Between and just above the eyebrows. **VII.** Just above the top of the head.

Begin as before, stretching, sitting, letting everything empty into your hara as you breathe out...all the way into the bottom of the void...and rise all the way up into that place where it is all one at the top of the breath...and empty back into the Tao at the very bottom.

Up to this point we have been using our breath as a vehicle as we move from state to state, but the fact is these states are continuous. The Tao does not stop being the Tao when we are up visiting the One. Nor does the One ever stop being One. Feel how constant they are...how the rising up the back continues even as you breathe out...and how the settling down the front continues to fall like a light golden snow even as you breathe in.

Feel both the rising and the settling at the same time...and both the Tao and the One. Feel where you are feeling this from...a place midway between the rising and the settling...a place midway between the Tao and the One...a point in the center of your chest, inside, in the center of your heart center...your most personal place.

Feel how deep inside that place is...and what vulnerability there is around it. It is your most individual place. It is you. And feel how whatever vulnerability, and guardedness, and past hurt surround it and shut it in, it can all be let go and emptied into the Tao. Let it all empty into the Tao as you breathe out. Everything empties into the Tao. And as you breathe in feel how much more open that place can become, how much love there is in it waiting to open out.

The Heart Chakra

The heart chakra is midway between the first chakra and the crown chakra. It is the center of the seven chakras. It has an outside (on our chest) and an inside (the deepest point inside). Love, the opening of this chakra, is when that which is inside connects to that which is outside. As we grow up, hurt accumulates from all the times we have felt abandoned or betrayed, when our hearts had been open to love and those of others had not. It becomes more and more difficult and threatening to let this chakra open. In Bodywork Tantra we learn to let this chakra open without any expectations (unconditional love). It is in being open that the heart chakra finds its true strength.

Because it has both an inside and an outside, this chakra has two pairs of meridians associated with it - Heart/Small Intestine and Circulation/Triple Heater.

The Heart meridian starts in the armpit and runs out the inside of the arm to the little finger. It connects to the Small Intestine meridian which runs up the back of the arm, across the shoulder blade and ends in front of the ear.

Their primary function is assimilation into the center. Traditionally they are related to the element fire, the color red, youth and joy. These are the meridians of the inside. The Heart is king and relates to our central control (and to meditation). In some schools of shiatsu the Heart meridian is not touched because it is sacred.

The Heart meridian has to do with the assimilation of love into our center and the Small Intestine meridian, the assimilation of other nutrients.

Heart 1. In the middle of the armpit.

Small Intestine 18. The depression under the cheek directly below the outer corner of the eye. **19.** The indentation just in front of the middle of the ear.

Stand, feet about twelve inches apart, knees not locked, back straight, shoulders relaxed. Breathe out...everything settling and emptying into the Tao. Breathe in...everything rising up the back... Focus on the rising. Feel how even as you breathe out you continue to feel that rising. It is continuous. Feel what is happening to each side of that rise. To each side there is a counter current flowing down the back. Focus on that counter current. It starts to the inside of the eyes, comes up over the top of the head, and flows all the way down the back, down the backs of the legs to the feet. Feel it flowing all the way down like water running off your back. And there is another flow down the sides of your body. Feel how it starts to the sides of your eyes, and flows down the sides of your head and neck and under your shoulder blades and through your hips and all the way down the sides of your legs to your feet. And there is another that starts just under your eyes. Feel how it flows all the way down your front, on down the fronts of your legs. Feel all three of these currents flowing from your head, flow down back, sides and front, all the way down to your feet...and feel how, from the toes and the bottom of the feet, all three flow up to the area around the heart. Feel them flowing all the way up the insides of your legs, all the way up to your heart. All three of these flows that begin in your head end in your heart.

Hold your arms out in front of you without twisting or locking them. Feel how there are three currents that start in the area around the heart and flow out to your hands. Feel all three flowing all the way out the insides of your arms, all the way out your fingers. And feel how they flow back up the backs of your arms, up through your shoulders and neck, all the way back up to your face. All three of these flows that begin in your heart end in your head.

Be aware of your heart and your head at the two ends of all these flows. Be aware of the inside of your heart and the inside of your head, your soul and your spirit, the two poles of all these flows that create and maintain the life of your body. These are the Two that are born out of the One. As you become aware of these two poles, and all the flows polarized between them, feel how your body starts to move, ever so slightly, a dance between these two that never touch. Enjoy the dance. It is your body.

Heart And Mind

When I first read the statement by Lao Tzu, I assumed that the basic rising of the yang and the falling of the yin were the Two born out of the One. Then as I worked more with the heart center meditation, I considered expanding the definition to encompass the outside (yang) and the inside (yin). And then I looked again at my meridian charts and saw how all the meridian pairs do have their yin end near the heart, and their yang end in the head. I had already begun to see the meridians as polarized forms of the energies in the chakras and now I saw how they are polarized between our heart center and the center in our head. The heart center is often cited as the seat of our "soul." In contrast what is centered in the head would then be our "spirit." The One gives birth to the Two. The soul is that which is individual within the universal, and the spirit, that which is universal within the individual. These are the most basic centers of the Yin and the Yang within us. And the meridian pairs polarized between them each carry one of the basic functions of our life force necessary to create and maintain our physical bodies. Where the pairs appear (or can be accessed) on our body relates to their function.

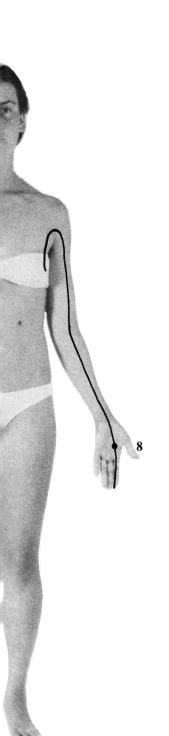

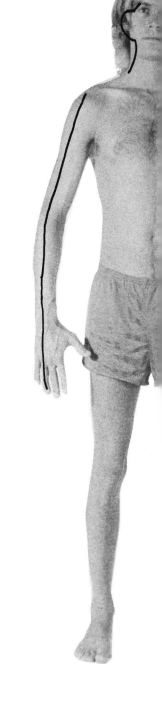

The Circulation meridian begins on the breast and runs out the midline of the inside of the arm ending on the middle finger. It connects to the Triple Heater meridian which runs up the midline up the back of the arm and ends on the outer corner of the eye brow.

The function of these meridians are protecting and moving out from the center. They, too, are related to fire, youth, the color red, and joy. The Circulation meridian has to do with our main circulation and the Triple Heater with our terminal circulation and the maintenance of our body warmth. It also has to do with the lymphatic system.

These are the meridians of the surface. The point between the breasts, the surface of the heart chakra, is related to the Circulation meridian.

Circulation 8. In the middle of the palm under the space between the middle and ring fingers.

Sit...back straight...shoulders relaxed...everything settling and emptying into your hara as you breathe out...and rising up your back as you breathe in...a wave spreading out to all parts of your body...and all those parts settle and empty into the Tao as you breathe out...everything empties into the Tao...and rises up into the One...the emptying and rising are continuous...and the Tao and the One...and in the middle is the center of your heart center...And inside your head is another center. These are the Two- the soul and the spirit. Focus on the Two, on how they move ever so slightly, without ever becoming closer or farther apart. The Yin and the Yang. Feel all the flows - down the back and legs...and back up to the heart...out arms...and back up to the head...Feel how all these flows are polarized between the Two...How, between them, they create and maintain your body. What a beautiful creation it is. And everything about your body, every strength and weakness, its beauty and its pleasures are creations of your soul and your spirit. And as a creation it is a work of art that has its own unique completeness. Feel its wholeness. And the center of that wholeness in your hara, just below your navel. What strength there is in that center. And there is another center in front of the heart. And one on the forehead - the third eye. The Two gives birth to the Three. These are the three centers that you face the world with - body...heart...and mind. Feel all three...your strength...your love...and your clarity.

The Navel Chakra

Our body center is just below the navel. It is the center of our physical body and its strength. In the area around it, the hara, each of the twelve meridians has its own area where the level of strength in that particular meridian can be felt and augmented (tonified). The Stomach/Spleen are the meridian pair associated with this chakra. The area used for diagnosing and strengthening the spleen meridian itself is around the navel, the center of the hara, an area associated with the earth (in China the earth is the center).

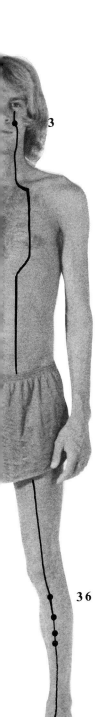

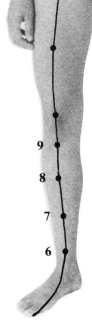

The Stomach meridian begins under the eyes and runs all the way down the front to end in the second toe. It is connected to the Spleen meridian which begins on the side of the big toe and runs up the inside of the legs to end in the chest. Spleen may be a mistranslation for pancreas whose functions in aiding digestion are associated with this meridian.

The main function of this pair is to provide our body its physical nurturance. It is traditionally connected to the earth element. The color is yellow; the time of life, maturity; and the emotional state; obsesssive thinking or worrying.

These are the meridians of the front. We go out in front of ourselves to get food. Food comes from the earth and is both our continuing connection to the earth and the source of our physical strength.

Being the meridians of the front these have to do with psychologically being out in front of ourselves in obsessions and worrying, probable indications (and causes) of imbalances in these meridians.

The stomach meridian has to do with the passageway of food through our body and the spleen (or pancreas) with the digestive juices and processes.

Stomach 3. On a line directly below the pupil, level with the base of the nose. **36.** Almost up to where attachments close the groove alongside the tibia, one finger breadth outside a slight protuberance on the tibia.

Spleen 6. 3 body inches above the tip of the medial malleolus (This and the following three points are close under the shinbone). **7.** In the depression 3 body inches above spleen 6. **8.** In the depression 4 body inches above spleen 7. **9.** In the depression 3 body inches above spleen 8 on a level with the tuberosity of the Tibia.

Begin again...sitting - back straight, shoulders relaxed...settling into the hara as you breathe out...rising up the back as you breathe in...emptying all the way into the bottom of the breath....rising all the way up at the top...and the settling and the rising...and the Tao and the One are continuous and you are in the middle....in the very center of your heart center...feel the distance to the surface.... How many times has the way into that center opened and closed! How many have you taken into that place...And feel the distance from the center of your mind to your third eye. Is it any greater or less than the distance from the center of the heart to the outside?...And feel the distance from the tips of your fingers and toes to the center below your navel...There are times when these distances seem so great that to travel would be going through a mountain...and other times when they have been as close as another's hand in your hand...Feel those distances disappear as your three centers on the surface open...Feel the balance between the three...Be aware of the whole area around each - the hara, the chest, and the head...and where these areas interface...Feel the point midway between the body center and the heart center, in the solar plexus. This is the center of the connection between body and heart, the center of our power, the center of our actions, our deeds. And the center between our heart center and mind center...Our throat center is the center of our words. Our words and our deeds are the Ten Thousand that are born out of the Three. Our deeds realize the balance between our strength and our love. Our words realize the balance between our love and clarity. Feel the balance, now, and, how, if your heart is not open, your deeds become dominated by a drive for power...and your words come out of your head. Open your heart even more. It can enter into your actions along with your strength...and into your words along with your thought. Feel the center in your solar plexus where strength and love combine.... Action in which both combine is true power...Feel the center in your throat where love and clarity combine...Speech in which both combine is true speech.

The Power Chakra

Midway between the navel chakra and the heart chakra, the power chakra is the center of our will and our acts. It is the third chakra. The first, the Tao, is energy in its pure potential state. The second, the navel center, is the place of our physical strength, our reserve of strength. This third is that strength put into action, which, when it is combined with our love from the fourth chakra becomes true power. When the love is absent it is the power of greed, of anger and rage.

These first chakras relate to the three meridian pairs of the legs; the power chakra to the Gall Bladder/Liver.

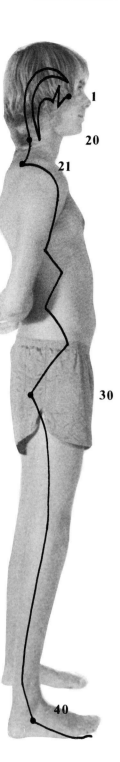

The Gall Bladder meridian starts to the outside corner of the eyes and runs down the sides of the body. It connects to the liver meridian which comes up the inside of the legs and ends in the chest.

The function of these meridians is the distribution and utilization of our physical energy. Traditionally these meridians are related to the element wood, to blue-green, to birth and to anger.

These are the meridians of the side. They are related to decision making (do I go this way or this way?).

Seeing the relationship between decision making, power and anger can help our understanding of these meridians. If we are powerless in our lives, if we don't have the power to make major decisions and/or have not learned, when appropriate, to surrender with love, anger results. An inability to let go of this often shows up in the right side of the back, around the shoulder blades and in the shoulders (where we force ourselves to hold back our desire to strike out), areas related to Gall Bladder/Liver.

Gall Bladder 1. On temple adjacent to outer corner of eye. **20.** In the largest hollow under the occiput. **21.** The middle point between the base of the neck and the end of the shoulder. **30.** In the large indentation on the hip. **40.** In the depression below and in front of the external malleolus.

Sit as before. Get in touch with the settling and the Tao...with the Tao and the rising...with the rising and the One.... Feel how the One becomes the Two that are deep inside your heart and your head (your soul and your spirit)...and how these two between them create your body as the Two become the Three- the three centers with which you face the world- body, heart and mind. Feel the balance between these three, and how between them they create the ten thousand deeds and words-between your body center and heart center- the center of your deeds- deeds that realize the balance between your strength and love....and between your heart and mind centers- the center of your words-words that realize the balance between your love and your clarity. Feel how throughout your life the balancing of these has been a continuing process, how there have been deeds that have come out of imbalance, out of anger or a drive for power, things you have done that you are still ashamed of. And how there have been words that have come out of imbalance, when your heart was closed to others, words that you have said and are still ashamed of. And all the deeds and words that can still fill you with shame, they are still out in front of you, between you and others. Breathe out, let them all empty back into the Tao, all the way into the bottom of the void. And as you breathe in and feel the rising, feel how balanced the centers of body, heart and mind can be, how your acts and words can fully realize your strength, and your love and your clarity. And there are things that you have done and said (and will do and say) that fill you with pride. Feel how they too are all out in front of you. And as you breathe out, let them, too, empty into the Tao. Let all 10,000 empty into the Tao, and the Three, and the Two, and the One. Let everything empty into the Tao.

The Throat Chakra

Midway between the heart chakra and the third eye, this chakra is where the energy of both is combined in our words, in our communication and compassion. If the heart chakra's love is cut off from this center our words become discompassionate and cold. If our mind's clarity is cut off our words can be full of feeling, but confused and unclear. Because this chakra and our power chakra are the chakras through which we go outside of ourselves in our ten thousand words and deeds, these are the chakras of our everyday life. The Throat Chakra is related to Lung/Large Intestine.

The Third Eye and the Senses

In the preceding we saw that the three meridian pairs of the legs are related to our first three chakras and all have to do with our physical strength- its potential, its presence and its manifestation in action.

The three meridian pairs of the arms are related to the next two chakras and have to do with the inside, its connection to the surface, and the interchange between the inside and the outside.

Every chakra has a meridian pair associated with it except the third eye. The senses, which are also energy pathways, are to the third eye what the meridians are to the other chakras.

Each sense can be divided into an outgoing (yang) and a receiving (yin). This is the differance between looking and seeing, or listening and hearing, etc. In the unpolarized energy of the third eye perception is not divided but is based on the unity between the perceiver and the perceived.

The Lung meridian begins in the corner of the chest and runs out the inside of the arm to the thumb. It connects to the Large Intestine meridian which begins in the first finger, runs up the back of the arm, and ends near the base of the nostril.

Their primary function is to govern the interchange between outside and inside. They are traditionally identified with the element metal; the color white; old age; and grief.

These are the meridians of the outside and have to do with forming boundaries. The skin is traditionally associated with them.

Lung 1. Between the first and second ribs 1 body inch below the middle of the clavicle. **2.** In the depression below acromial extremity of the clavicle. **3.** On the medial aspect of the upper arm on the radial side of the biceps, 3 body inches below the axillary fold. **5.** In the fold of the elbow inside the tendon when you make a fist. **6.** On radial aspect of forearm 7/12ths of the way from the wrist to the elbow. **9.** Indentation below the base of the thumb in wrist.

Large Intestine 4. On the middle of the second metacarpal bone where the muscle mounds up when the thumb and forefinger are brought close together. **8.** 4 body inches below L.I. 11. **9.** 3 body inches below L.I. 11. **10.** 2 body inches below L.I. 11. **11.** In the depression at the end of the fold when the elbow is bent 90 degrees. **20.** In the small grooves just outside the widest point of the nostrils.

In China the meridian pairs have been traditionally classified with the elements and their associated qualities and processes. In the table opposite these traditional associations are combined with the chakras as they are related to each meridian pair in this book. These associations do not always correspond to the way elements are associated with chakras in the various Indian systems. In India the elements are seen on a scale from coarser to finer. Since there is an emphasis on rising up from lower to higher, the coarsest element, the earth, is assigned to the lowest chakra. In China, however, the elements are seen not as substances, but as transformational processes in a continual cycle, in which all are essential, and none have a higher or lower place.

The organization into three levels on the opposite page corresponds to our three basic centers. The 'levels of creation' derived in this book from Lao Tzu's quote are also incorporated in the chart. For ease of reference I am including the quote below and a brief summary of how it is applied to the meridian pairs and the chakras in this book.

> The Tao gives birth to the One ...
> The One gives birth to the Two ...
> The Two gives birth to the Three ...
> And the Three to the Ten Thousand

The relationship between our different states and levels of energy is that of creation itself. The rise of energy up the midline of the back (kundalini) is the birth of the One out of the Tao (the undifferentiated, the 'mother of all beings'). And down its paired meridian down the front everything empties and returns to the Tao. The Two born out of the One are our soul (the individual in the universal) and our spirit (the universal in the individual). These are the yin and yang poles of our meridian pairs (each has one end in the chest and one in the head). Each meridian pair carries one basic function of our life force. All living beings, even one-celled organisms, have the same set of functions...and the same meridians. Where the meridian appears on the body relates to its function. The meridian pairs are polarized between our soul and spirit to create and maintain our physical body. On our bodies there are three basic centers (the Three born out of the Two), the centers of body, heart and mind. Between our body center and heart center there is the center of our deeds which realize the balance (or lack of it) between our body's strength and heart's love. Between our heart center and mind center is the center of our words which realize the balance between our heart's love and our mind's clarity. Our deeds and words are the 10,000 that are born out of the Three. Our senses are energy pathways with both yin (looking, etc.) and yang (seeing, etc.). In our third eye perception is not polarized but unified (its perception is based on identity with the perceived). This parallels the relationship between the other chakras and their related meridians. There is a similar relationship between our mind center (the inside) and our thoughts, which are also energy pathways with a yang (searching the past) and yin (remembering) polarization. And just as our senses create the space around us our thoughts create the time around us.

Energy Pathways Centered in the Head

ASPECT	time	space	God
FUNCTION	thought	perception	creation
MEANS	memory	the senses	creation
CHAKRA	sixth(inner)	sixth(outer)	seventh
LOCATION	inside head	the third eye	crown
LEVEL OF CREATION	the Two	the Three	the One
CENTER	spirit	mind	universe
ENERGY	knowledge	clarity	unity

Pathways of the Arms (Yin/Yang)

ASPECT	inside	surface	outside
MERIDIAN PAIR	Heart/Sm. Intestine	Circulation/TripleH.	Lung/L. Intestine
FUNCTION	central control	protection	interchange
MEANS	assimilation	circulation	boundaries
ELEMENT	fire	fire	metal
TISSUE	blood vessels	blood vessels	skin
SENSE ORGAN	tongue	tongue	nose
BODY FLUID	sweat	sweat	mucous
EMOTION	joy	joy	grief
EXPRESSION	laughing	laughing	weeping
COLOR	red	red	white
TASTE	bitter	bitter	pungent
SEASON	summer	summer	autumn
STAGE OF LIFE	youth	youth	old age
CHAKRA	fourth(inner)	fourth(outer)	fifth
LOCATION	inside chest	chest	throat
LEVEL OF CREATION	the Two	the Three	the 10,000
CENTER	soul	heart	words
ENERGY	love	feeling	communication

Pathways of the Legs (Yang/Yin)

ASPECT	back	front	sides
MERIDIAN PAIR	Bladder/Kidney	Stomach/Spleen	Gall Bladder/Liver
FUNCTION	purification	nourishment	distribution
MEANS	elimination	digestion	planning
ELEMENT	water	earth	wood
TISSUE	bones	fat or flesh	muscles,ligaments
SENSE ORGAN	ears	mouth	eyes
BODY FLUID	urine	saliva	tears
EMOTION	fear	obsession, worry	anger
EXPRESSION	groaning	singing	shouting
COLOR	black	yellow	green(blue)
TASTE	salty	sweet	sour
SEASON	winter	late summer	spring
STAGE OF LIFE	death	maturity	birth
CHAKRA	first	second	third
LOCATION	perineum	below navel	solar plexus
LEVEL OF CREATION	the Tao	the Three	the 10,000
CENTER	the void	body	deeds
ENERGY	potential	strength	power

A NOTE ON DIAGNOSIS

In my studies I was taught a form of meridian diagnosis based on feeling the 'kyo' (low energy) and 'jitsu' (excess energy) in the meridians. The relationship between the kyo and jitsu was illustrated by drawing a circle (like a clock where each hour represents one meridian) or a balloon. Wherever there is an indention in one portion (kyo in one meridian) there is a related bulge (jitsu) in another portion. Jitsu, with its obvious tension and symptoms, is easy to locate. Kyo is hidden. When a jitsu area is pressed it presses back, whereas a kyo area may be felt as a plank-like stiffness protecting some underlying weakness. In general the excess energy in the jitsu areas can be released by movement and stretching, and the kyo areas, re-energized by steady holding. Ideally these areas could be balanced by maintaining the mother hand on the kyo area and working with the other hand on the jitsu area. The basis of oriental medicine is that it is these imbalances in our meridians lead to disease. If we balance the energy in the meridians we prevent disease and maintain health.

In acupuncture meridian diagnosis is done by feeling the pulses in the wrist. In my classes I was taught to feel for the kyo and jitsu in the hara and the back, and for differences in the quality of the different meridian stretches. What we are feeling in the hara is the immediate condition of the meridians, their balance at this moment, and the relative strength of each meridian. What we feel in the various meridian areas of the back is their chronic conditions, what is called in this book, their holding.

In Bodywork Tantra, the more we incorporate work with chakras and engage our own chakras, the more we can 'be' with a person; the more connected we are to that person, the more we are 'led' to those places that need attention, and the more we stay as long and with as much pressure as needed. Treatment is diagnosis. And to the degree our moves are determined by a preconceived diagnosis and our ability to respond intuitively and spontaneously is curbed, diagnosis can be counter productive.

The patterns of this book emphasize working on the whole body. Every meridian pair is worked, and if we stay connnected and open to be called where needed, we will be facilitating that person's meridians' return to balance. The body's energy system is a self-healing mechanism. Any attention to the meridians and chakras encourages them to return to balance. Our goal is not to 'zap' someone, to heal them with our energy, but to be with them and stay empty. The emptier (in the sense of being in the Tao) we are, the more effective will our presence be. And if we are empty and holding someone in two places, whatever is released with the one hand is free to go through us and out the other to where needed. As we work we will become more aware of what meridians are releasing or filling the most. This awareness, our diagnosis, can watch over the work and tell us, when we return to the same needy meridian in a different position, to be attentive.

Our staying empty is our greatest (and only) protection from picking up any negativity during our work. To the degree our ego is involved, to the degree we are attached to proving what great healers we are, to the degree we are trying to do something to someone, to that degree we are in danger of creating a negative reaction in ourselves. And that danger is compounded to the degree we believe that others can dump their negative energy on us, to the degree we believe we have to shake the person's energy off our hands, to the degree we believe any energy is negative. Tension is energy blocked. And all energy is divine.

And when we are not empty, when our ego is involved, when we are trying to do something to someone, our work will be less effective, because our trying is bound to create resistance (as is any fear we have).

To stay empty may sound difficult at first, but one of the beauties of Bodywork Tantra is, that the more you practice, the easier you will find it to connect and work from that empty place.

Being empty in this sense does not mean to completely shut off your mind. Your knowledge of the different meridians and their relationships to specific conditions can play a part in the process. You can choose a particular sequence of moves according to what you feel that person needs. i.e. If someone has a lot of problems with colds and allergies choose positions in which you can pay attention to the Lung and Large Intestine meridians. But at the same time work with the whole body and stay wherever needed and go wherever called. You can monitor this and, according to your own growing awareness of that person's imbalances, add positions and work accordingly.

At the end of a session people often ask what you found wrong with them. Be careful. If a person is not aware of how, when we talk about meridians we are talking about a general function, and not just the organ related to that function; and you tell that person you felt something wrong in his liver meridian, he may program himself for liver failure. So powerful is the mind.

Many people may come to you expecting you to fix them. The trouble with the doctor-patient model is that it prevents the 'patient' from becoming aware of his own power. In Bodywork Tantra, the most we can do for others is to get them in touch with their own healing energy. Most people walk around with so little awareness of what beings of energy they are. By being there with them, we can become witnesses to their discovery of their being. And that moment is love. And if we needed a model from outside Bodywork Tantra to approximate what we do, it would be that of lover-lover.

AN AUTOBIOGRAPHY OF ENERGY

I have found in my own life a continuing relationship between a developing bodywork tantra practice and a practice of tantric lovemaking. One feeds the other. It is one practice.

In order to help the reader reach his fullest potential in his own practice, I feel I shouldn't end this book without saying something about this other side of the practice.

And rather than just saying 'X happens and it feels great,' I think it would help the reader more if I explore what brought me to the point where X could happen; and in the process reach a greater clarity about the different forms of energy we experience in our practice and in our lives (which is the subject of this book).

Looking back through my life for prototypes or sources of what I experience in tantra, I see recurring three basic states: awe, rapture, and clarity. These interestingly correlate with our three-fold division: body, heart and mind. Awe is the feeling in our body when we suddenly find ourselves in the presence of something totally beyond our understanding. Goosebumps tingle over our whole body. Rapture is the opening of our heart to what is outside. Clarity is a feeling of being in total light. In Tantra these three feelings naturally flow together into ecstasy (enlightenment).

It has not always been that way. I remember early experiences of awe accompanied with fear and terror triggered by something as simple as a curtain moving in the wind as I lay in bed in the dark trying to go asleep- God coming to destroy the world? In my grandfather's pentecostal church I had been told over and over that He would. And I lay in bed and prayed He wouldn't, that I would not 'die before I wake.' For, though I had felt the 'call,' I could not 'open up my heart' and walk up to be 'saved' (and deny my mother and all the other non-pentecostals marked for destruction).

One place where I could open my heart was about as far away from people as I could get, out on the Puget Sound tideflat, so far out that the houses and all their conflicts were just a thin line smoke rose from, as I chased seagull after seagull, following their rise up in ever widening circles, or built castle after castle with a concentration so total not even the knowledge of their certain destruction by the tide's rising could disturb.

Rapture is the natural state of the infant. It is only when his heart's openness is not met by the openness of those around him that he begins to shut down.

A later memory is that of singing when I was sixteen, driving my car around and around, making up my own words to some popular song whose words and tune I could never quite get. And I remember the writing of my first poem, a Dylan Thomasish rhapsody to the moon. And later, when a poem would come to me on its own, it would sometimes be accompanied with a rapture and a clarity that felt like it was being written with light itself. But they didn't come that way as often as I would like.

But I could sometimes experience similar states reading other's poems, or looking at paintings, or listening to music. And I would take long walks in the woods to suddenly find myself in a place where I felt such a wholeness...such awe...something I would feel again climbing a temple ruin in Mexico or Peru...or a shinto shrine in Japan...or stepping out onto the beach at the ocean.

And it was in the ocean that I first learned that this awe, and the rapture, and the clarity that comes out of it could be part of a regular practice. For two years I lived at Stinson Beach and every day would go down body surfing in the ocean. Northern California waters are cold. But I soon learned that if I focused my concentration on the waves, on their power and brightness, I could feel it as energy which kept my body warm...and when a wave broke that carried me all the way up -what rapture! And what clarity standing up again in the middle of that frothing bright water, striding back out for the next wave.

And after living in Mexico City, three years away from the ocean, I came back. Climbing down a gully, I began to feel an awe drawing me to it even before I saw it- the whole sea bathed in light. I sat out on the limb of a tree fallen out over that bright water. And as a wave rose up words rose up and came out as a complete sentence in a language I had never heard before. And then another wave - the voice, the words of another rose up and came out my mouth. Each wave's voice and words different (all those who have drowned at sea?)... And whatever each needed to say seemed totally completed as each wave broke...And then I saw two seals, their heads out of the waves, and wondered what they were doing watching me when, all of a sudden, loud and clear:

"YOUR VOICE IS EVERYBODY'S VOICE"

In the silence that followed was a completeness nothing could ever take away from or add to. But there still seemed one more thing that had to be done. Maybe just because I didn't know what else to do with all that energy. Or maybe because the spiritual is even closer to the sexual than we realize. I took off all my clothes and, the sun shining on me, came into the ocean. There was none of that loss of energy I sometimes feel afterwards. The sea, if anything, was more radiant than before.

Tantra takes many forms. And that experience was no less tantric than those that come later. To ejaculate or not to ejaculate is not the issue. The issue is how to open up our connection to others and experience the freedom of our connected energies. And the problem with ejaculation is it usually does get in the way and, with its moment of pleasure, limit us. And even before it happens, if our consciousness is directed towards it as a goal, it limits and keeps us from being there with the other.

My first awareness of this was when I was in college and looked back at those few furtive moments that, preceded with such longing, ended so suddenly. I realized that in none of them had I been aware of what the girl might be feeling. I started to make a conscious effort to hold back my coming...or if I couldn't do that...to go on from it to further comings...which was not difficult for I had always had a lot of energy. So much so that one recurring terror in Junior High School was that the teacher would make me stand up to answer a question when I had an erection. Which seemed to be more often the case than not. And there has been only one time in my life when it hasn't responded when I wanted it to (as opposed to all the times it responded when I hadn't wanted it to). And that was when I was at my lowest point - my wife of seven years had just run off with a friend of mine and taken my twin daughters...and I had followed them to New York and saw there was no way I could get them back...and I set up house with a wild readhead who had the most disconcerting habit of everytime we made love, if I stopped moving for just a moment (which I had to do to keep from coming), she would go into a coma which five minutes later she would come out of with no idea what happened or where she'd been...and after a month of that we had just broken up when I met a girl in a bar and walked around for hours, listening to her expound on Wilhelm Reich and what kind of orgasm a man should have (I had no idea what she was talking about) and when I finally got her into my little bed in my crummy little lower East Side flat and she had all her clothes off, my body just wasn't there...I don't know where it was...but it wasn't there...and she walked away in disgust at having found another man unable to live up to her expectations. That was the lowest point.

But I recovered. And as soon as I got back to San Francisco I met the woman I was to live with the next twenty years and poems to Venus ('on the horizon the hour I was born') began to pour out

How I am drawn back into that dark
once more
to stand on the shore
before the mystery at the prow of Venus's bark

as it scrapes sand and foamy dress thrown off
she steps out.
How I am drawn back to that spot
I heard, running towards her new flowery dress, her cry and laugh

Oh beauty born in the deep of night
Oh beauty born of sexual delight.

But even in that first year of our love there was some tension as a poem that came out when we moved up to Stinson Beach reveals

Sanosa como la mar
esta la nina
Ay, Dios! quien le hablaria?

When she rode in on the wave and walked back smiling "It's
    beautiful. You really ride on top of the wave." I felt
    as good as if I had ridden in

and when after several failures trying to 'get right there
    where the wave breaks' as she said a wave carried me all
    the way in on top of it and I walked back to her she
    looked as happy as if she had ridden in

but when that 'right wave' I had waited so long for broke
    over me and the board broke under me against my balls and
    I jumped up in pain with only the top of the board in my
    hand in the froth beside me holding up the bottom she
    screamed
            "You broke it and I never got my turn again! You
    hogged it! You're so selfish! You would never let me have
    my turn and now you broke it!"
                            and all the way up the shore
    all the way up to the men's showers she ran after me
    waving the bottom shouting riding on top of the crest
    of the wave of her anger

I feel in it a celebration of love and energy (even the energy of her anger which I wasn't always able to celebrate...or run away from). But I also feel in that sudden breaking of the boogy board (which I wasn't going to need anyway once I learned to body surf) something of what I feel when I come too soon, even if I am able to go on and come again, as I still almost always did. (But years later she complained about being my 'sex slave' that first year.)

But things got better when I read Masters and Johnson and discovered the clitoris. The clitoris is such a household word today that it is hard to believe there was a time when men didn't know what it was there for. But I guess there were a lot of others in the same boat. Discovering the clitoris opened up a whole new world. I found that if I could get over my initial fear and excitement first coming in, if I could cross that bridge, and focus on her pleasure, that I could feel her energy beginning its rise. Once I was locked into the rising wave of her energy, and kept my concentration there, I couldn't come until I felt her go all the way over the top. It was beautiful.

Years later when I had my first experience with a woman who had multiple orgasms I discovered I could ride over each wave and come with her on the last wave.

And years later I discovered there didn't have to be a last wave.

This feeling of riding and being connected to another's waves of energy was what I would start feeling with everybody when I did shiatsu.

I was forty and had never had a massage myself when, at a hot springs (The Geysers), I went up to a woman I was attracted to and asked her if she would like a massage. She said yes. And when she could feel how little I knew about what I was doing, she had me lie down and showed what to do to her. I didn't make the sexual connection I had in mind, but she gave me something more important. When we got back to the city she taught me Esalen. I hadn't yet got around to buying a table (I had set up a padded board in my hot tub to massage people in the water- what I called 'wassage') when she practiced on me the shiatsu she was learning from Ohashi and I knew that's what I wanted to do.

I started studying with the zen priest, Reuho Yamada, at the temple he had specifically set up for shiatsu. Learning and practicing shiatsu effected profound changes in me. Up to then I had been becoming more and more cut off from others, insulated within my marriage and my house and my conception of the natural superiority being a poet gave me. But now I was able to come close to others...to be with them and accept them as they are...without judgment...to feel how everyone is beautiful and complete within themselves.

I would make regular trips to Skagg's Springs, a place where I could always find people around the pools to practice on. Occasionally it would be a woman who opened up to a more intimate connection, something I seemed to need at that time of my life, still not yet having recovered from the deprivations and rejections of adolescence ('Every one you miss you're one behind the rest of your life,' my stepfather, a career navy man, used to say). And one night at Skagg's Springs (which has since been buried under the waters of a reservoir) a poem came to me in a dream

SNAKE

Snake shakes
its diamonds in the water

and all our loves
shine and come out to play

Snake shakes
its diamonds in the water

and all we have
shimmers and flows away

Snake shakes
its diamonds in the water

But at the same time shiatsu was bringing me to those who enjoyed helping me make up what I had missed so, it was showing me that it wasn't that important, that the connection I made doing the shiatsu was complete and sufficient unto itself; that I could be with women (and men) and feel a loving connection that was free of desire. And I learned to respect the moment and the trust people put in me too much to ever use shiatsu as a means. I came to end each session with open arms...to let go.

And one morning, very early, I went down to a pool and found a woman sitting in it. I asked her if she would like a shiatsu and started working on her right in the water. When I finished she turned her head from side to side and said she hadn't been able to move it like that since she had been in an accident. She said she could feel healing coming through my hands. I thanked her, and my joy at hearing what she said stayed with me as I strode up the side of a mountain, up into a circle of trees at the top whose limbs were filled with light. Such awe. God is here. I dropped to my knees. He bent down and lifted me up...and walked at my side...and led me along a stream. But when we came to where the stream's bed tangled below in brush, I saw an easier path down the gully's side. I asked "Which way do I go?" He said "Whichever way you go I am with you." Words that have never left me.

And back by the pool I sat on the bank and saw how the pool, and the children splashing in the water, and the trees; and the birds singing in the branches, how we are all sitting in His hand.

And again at another low point in my life (I had just left a therapy session with my wife where I finally had the acknowledgement pried out of me that there was no way I could go back to her), a point at which I felt an absolute powerlessness, and I was lying on the table of a friend who was doing Reichian work with me, tears in my eyes, saying over and over 'I have no power of my own'...'I have no power of my own,' a mantra at the deepest level of my being, when, just over my feet, I saw His huge face, as round and as bright as the sun, pouring golden light into my heart, filling me, who had no power.

And another time I felt that light pouring, this time from another direction. I was out on the dance floor of the Rajneesh Center in Munich where my Tantsu students had brought me. I had felt such love from my students in that first class there. And dancing I felt such awe that I should receive that much love. And golden light began to pour onto my head and shoulders...and poured and poured as I danced and danced...and I thought of my sweetie...and of all the love she gives me...and it poured more and more...and the whole time it was pouring I could feel my own energy rising up my back. The dance is the joining of the two.

Another time I felt both this pouring and rising in the middle of awe, was when I stepped back onto the campus of my alma mater, the University of Washington, after so many years away, and felt still in me the self that walked down that same path and sat in those classrooms. As I sat on the grass, all the selves I've ever lived as student or teacher came through me, one after the other.

And again, just this winter, a similar pouring and upwelling of the past as I sat and watched my son and the other competitors strutting on their bicycles, warming up for a free style contest - Tournament jousters in their bright colors...Aztec warriors in their feathers and flowers...

So many forms and movements that energy can take. There is no limit to it.

But I am getting ahead of myself. The rising up my back, which is such an integral part of all these experiences, had been being nurtured and developed in my practice of Sexual Tantra.

The first time I experienced this rising was when a woman I had just given a watsu to floated me in return. A powerful vibration started moving up my back. When I stood up in the pool it kept rising, straightening my back so. I later found that if I had someone hold my perineum, that that would set it off. I began to feel a similar rising up my back giving a watsu and wrote

THE WATER DANCE
Full Moon, July, 1983

If you happen to find your way into the warm pool at Harbin Hot
    Springs
and an old man with a white beard drifts up to your side
and, casually mentioning he comes up every weekend to teach
    the Shiatsu classes,
asks if you would like some in the water - 'watsu' he calls it
    "something I developed in the pool here...I like to practice
    it every chance I get..."
accept
and you will find yourself being floated
your neck in the crook of his arm your sacrum in his hand
as he rocks you back and forth...back and around...back into a
    world without sound...back into the waters of the womb
as he swirls and sways you the way dolphins play
as he stretches leg and arm and back every way water allows
or drapes your legs over his shoulders and lifts you clear of it
the way an old man plays with the daughters of creation
and sets you down astraddle his held out leg
so that the chakra in your perineum is held from below by his
    thigh
and your hara by one hand
and your lower back by the other
so that the energy locked in that bowl is free to rise all the
    way up your spine
and join that old man's
two intertwining taoist dragons soaring heavenward

Or
refuse.
Maybe he is just another lecherous old man
coming on
to all the pretty girls in the pool
"Thank you
I just want to be by myself..."
He
will find another
and another
and another
The sky is filled with dragons

Oh Lady of the Waters
no bluer pasture
could you have turned me out into...
How I love all these ladies
who pass through my arms
a splash and a wave
the flash of a tail
the look they turn to me with...
and though it has been two years
since I wrote my last poem

spiralling up from that dragon's head
it has not been a dry period
for I have been floating
my muse
and know one day
she may turn
and show me her face

And one night
someone floats me in return
and again I spiral up from that dragon's head
but this time I call Astarte and Serpent to help enter
   that world above
but it isn't until I call St. George (how could I have
   forgotten him?) and feel his straightness in my spine
that I am suddenly inside that light
and it is nothing like the streets and clouds of buildings
   I saw from below
but a continuous shining out to all directions
long fine spikes of light
the spines of a great sea urchin
each shining out whirling worlds and universes

and it is inside each of us

we are lighthouses
floating on a dark sea
lighting the way to each other

The above poem came to me the morning after I gave my first watsu to Valerie. She had seen a video of me giving a watsu at the Body Mind Spirit Festival six months earlier (at which time, she has since told me, she knew she would be with me) and had finally gotten around to coming up to Harbin. She began coming up more and more.

I found in Valerie a woman I could be completely myself with, a woman with whom I did not have to try to be other than whatever part of my self was ready to come up at that moment. And she found a like trust and safety in me. At the end of our first year together I wrote

TANTRA
for Valerie

I
She shimmies up the spine
   winds her legs around each vertabra
     and shimmers and shakes

And when she's up at the top
   she's still at the bottom
     She never stops

II
Tantra is as many sided
as heaven and earth
when a man has a woman
he can share everything with...
and when he remembers
the way mother
caught him masturbating
on a pile of dirty laundry
and walked away in silence
he tells her...
and when he enters
as vulnerable as that child
he tells her...
and when she melts around him
and he is a child
making love for the first time
in innocence and joy
he tells her...
and when
surrounded by her tenderness and love
the child grows into a man
who thrusts deeper and deeper
and she looks up
with all the power of a woman
and says 'Master'
there is nothing he cannot do or be -
a lion roaring
or a dragon swooping down
claws so sharp
they could tear her apart...
"I could tear you apart
but won't...
You open my heart so..."

III
It is beginning
It is rising together
eyes and bodies one
lightning and thunder
It is meeting the dragon on the mountaintop

It is continuing
It is moving together
eddies and swirls up the back
pebbles singing in the clear water
It is meeting the dragon in the river

It is arrival
It is coming together
from every single direction
one great wave that never breaks
It is meeting the dragon in the middle of the ocean

From almost the beginning with Valerie I started feeling the vibrations up my back while making love. The stronger they were, the less I would feel any need to ejaculate. I learned that if I got close to ejaculating, if I moved my attention up to my heart chakra and felt it opening, surrounding Valerie, the energy would start moving up my back. I have since read different books on Tantric and Taoist lovemaking. The traditional tantric books emphasize a greater sense of ritual. The taoists inject an element of fear with dire threats as to what will happen to you if you leak out or spill your energy. My own experiences with energy moving into and through me and out of me in so many ways makes it hard for me to conceptualize it as a limited quantity. And getting free of fear has been for me the key to Tantra. I feel I am not avoiding ejaculation out of fear, but because another kind of orgasm has been given me I can share with my partner over and over.

But it may be my experience is exceptional. And that others, if they want to develop their own practice need first to follow some method that either involves lying still (as some tantric books suggest) or developing a powerful lock on their muscles. Or it may be, as I'd rather think, that those who practice the Bodywork Tantra of this book will feel greater connections to others and movements of energy in their own bodies which can become the basis of a tantric sexual practice.

As our practice has unfolded, Valerie and I, who celebrated our marriage in a watsu wedding in the warm pool last year, have experienced more and more forms and movements of energy. Besides the rising up the back which we call S.O.'s (spiritual orgasms), I sometimes experience F.O.'s (flying orgasms) in which my whole body is flying, carried on slow, undulating waves completely different than the short fast waves of an S.O. There is no limit to the forms love takes. Sometimes I am completely surrounding Valerie. Sometimes I am completely inside her, feeling her orgasm from the inside. She is with me in so many ways. She says the S.O.s fill her and nourish her more than food. And, besides her regular orgasms, she has begun to have what she calls L. O.s (love orgasms), a sudden opening of her heart, a sweet shuddering which she might feel any place just looking at me, in a restaurant or wherever, which sets me off into an immediate S.O.

Underlyling the difference between an S.O. and an L.O. may be a basic difference between the way men and women experience Tantra: the man begins with the rising up out of the first chakra; and the woman with the heart's opening, an opening that descends to open her whole body. In meditation I experience the rise up the back as direct and forceful and yang; and the descent as yin, as slow as snow falling with an accompanying feeling of openness and letting go. Men and women experience both. It is a continuous cycle in everyone. But which place they can most easily enter into the cycle differs; and is complementary. When they join in Tantra they create a single cycle of their combined energies more complete than either could feel alone.

That once the cycle is joined, the connection is maintained even when separated, came home the other day as, alone on the beach, I watched Valerie walk towards me and felt such power grow that she began to blush and giggle and, in her joy, laugh in the bright waves dancing before me.

A Tantric Lovemaking practice and a Bodywork Tantra practice feed into and support one another. The S.O.s I sometimes have giving a watsu, or a tantsu, or just holding someone, keep getting stronger (And when Valerie steps into the pool and sees me having an S.O. with someone she smiles, sharing my enjoyment). The connection I celebrate with others in those moments is complete in itself. 'Tantra of the Loving Hug', I call it. I once started to set up workshops to teach it, but realized the Watsu classes themselves were the best way to get people into the space where they could share energy this way, the weekends often ending in a circle in the warm pool, our hearts open, vibrations rising up all our backs. It is beautiful. And there is no end to it.

CIRCLES CELEBRATING CONNECTION

A process in which you get in touch with and open your energy's flows and centers through stretching and meditation and then connect and celebrate them in circles with others.

The circles were developed to join and play with the energy being liberated in our Bodywork Tantra classes. This process was developed for the Harmonic Convergence ceremonies here at Harbin. Its reception encouraged me to offer it regularly to both students and non-students. It is complete in itself. What follows is a script for this process (including stage directions) with which you can lead groups of six or more people. If you have a larger group it can, after the meditation, break up into circles of 8 to 14. The participants can be wearing loose clothing to facilitate stretching. Allow up to 2 hours.

The Opening And The Stretches

Start with them standing in a large circle around you. Have each introduce themselves. Say

In this process we work with the flows and centers of energy in our own bodies and then connect them in circles. We start out with stretches to get in touch with the meridian flows. The meridians come in pairs. We are going to do one stretch for each pair. Each pair carries one function of the life force in our body. Where these pairs appear on our body relates to their function. For example, the Stomach/Spleen meridian pair appears on the front of our body. We go out in front of ourselves to get food. Enter into each of the following stretches gradually without straining yourself. As you breathe in hold the stretch, and as you breathe out settle a little deeper into it and feel the stretched meridians gradually let go and open. We will begin with the Lung and Large Intestine meridians which are the meridian pair of the outside and relate to the interchange between outside and inside.

Demonstrate this and the subsequent meridian pair stretches from page 76. After they finish the last stretch say

Keep your eyes closed and stand up. Be still for a moment and feel whatever movements of energy through your body these stretches have helped open and bring into your awareness. There is one flow that comes up over the top of your head and flows all the way down to your feet. Be aware of it to both sides of your spine flowing like water down your back. Feel how this flow returns up from the very bottom of your feet, up the insides of your legs, up to your chest. Be aware of another flow that begins to the outside corners of your eyes and flows all the way down your sides, down your feet..and back up the insides of your legs, up to your chest. And another flow beginning under your eyes, flowing down through your breasts, all the way down the front of your legs to your feet and back up the insides of your legs to your chest. All these flows that begin in your head, that flow down back, sides and front, return up the insides of your legs to end in your chest. Your head and your chest, the area around your heart, are the two poles of these meridian pairs' flows.

Now hold your arms out in front of you. Feel the flows from your chest out the insides of your arms to your thumb and fingers...and feel how these flows return back up the backs of your arms, up the neck to the face. The heart and head are the two poles of all these meridian flows. These flows that create and maintain the life of our bodies are polarized between the heart and the head, the yin and the yang. Lower your arms, keep your eyes closed. We have other energy pathways in addition to our meridian pairs. Our senses too have a yin and a yang aspect. When I tell you to open your eyes I want you to look around and find whatever point is farthest away from you. Open your eyes and look. Close your eyes. Now, without looking for anything in particular, open your eyes and see whatever is in front of you. Close your eyes again. When you look for something that is the yang of sight. When you see without looking that is the yin of sight. All our senses are pathways with yin and yang aspects. Listen and hear. Our thoughts are also pathways. Take a moment to search for the most distant moment in your past. Now let go of it and let whatever image will come up in your mind. The searching is yang and the letting happen is yin. And just as our meridian pairs create our physical bodies, our senses' pathways create the space around us and our thoughts create the time we exist in.

Each of these pathways is related to a particular center or chakra in our bodies. Focus your attention on your third eye. The senses are related to this chakra. Whatever you perceive with your third eye is without separation between you and what you perceive. In the pathways our energy is polarized. In the chakras it is unified and resonates to connect to other chakras, our own and others. We are going to do a meditation now which will help you open and feel some of the connections between your chakras. We will connect chakras on the levels on which they continue the creation cycle as described by Lao Tzu in the Tao Te Ching: The Tao gives birth to the one...The One gives birth to the Two...The Two gives birth to the Three...And the Three to the Ten Thousand.

The Creation Cycle Meditation

If you are used to it, sit in lotus; if not, sit in the most comfortable position you can which will help you keep your back straight. You can use a cushion if you want.

Sit with your back straight and your shoulders relaxed. Close your eyes.

> **The Tao gives birth to the one...**
> **The One gives birth to the Two...**
> **The Two gives birth to the Three...**
> **And the Three to the Ten Thousand...**

Take a deep breath and, as you let it all the way out, feel a letting go in your hara (abdomen). And a rising up your back as you breathe in. Continue feeling this as you breathe normal deep breaths. Feel that rising up your back as you breathe in as a wave spreading out to all parts of your body. And feel how all those parts let go and settle and empty into the hara as you breathe out. Be aware of any part that doesn't let go as much as the rest. That is where you are holding tension. Tension is blocked energy. The next time you breathe in fill that part even more...and let it go and settle and empty into the hara as you breathe out...

The whole area of the hara is a bowl around the base of the spine, the navel- the front, the sacrum- the back and the perineum between your legs- the bottom. As you breathe out let everything empty into that bowl.

At the very bottom of the breath the bowl itself empties into the point at the bottom- the first chakra. There our energy enters into the void - a state in which it is most powerful because it is pure potential. Stay there a little longer at the bottom of each breath. The deeper you let go into it the more powerful the rising up your back as you breathe in. That void is the Tao, the undifferentiated, the mother of all beings. And the rising up the back is the One being born out of the Tao. And the One is the crown chakra over your head, where you are one with everything...a world of pure light. Rise all the way up your back into that light. It is not a light seen, but a being light- a shining out to all sides. Stay being that light a moment and then let everything settle down your front slowly descending like snow falling, darkening as it empties into the Tao.

What you have felt rising up your back and settling down the front is continuous. We have used the breath as a vehicle to ride up and down. But the rising and settling are continuous. And the Tao and the One are continuous. And the continuous rising and the One and the settling and the Tao make one continuous circle. Feel where your awareness of that circle is centered- in the center of that circle. In the center of your chest. In the very center of your heart center. This is your most personal, individual place. Feel what vulnerability there is around your heart center, how your shoulders want to close in and protect it. The next time you breathe out let all that vulnerability and hurt and protectiveness settle and empty into the Tao.

Feel how open your heart center can be. And there is another center deep inside your head, your mind center. Focus on these two centers and feel whatever movement there is in your body from side to side. Feel how these two centers never come closer together and never move farther apart, but stay balanced- the yin and the yang. These are the Two that are born out of the One. Feel how they dance, polarizing between them all the meridians that create and maintain the life of your body. Your body is created in this dance of your heart and mind. Your soul and your spirit. What a beautiful creation your body is.

And your body has its own center just below your navel. And there is another center on the front of your chest- your heart chakra. And on the front of your head- your third eye. These are the Three born out of the Two, the three you face the world with, the centers of your strength, love and clarity. Feel what rocking forward movement there is as these three centers balance and dance.

Between your body center and your heart chakra, in the solar plexus is the center of your deeds, your actions, your will. Your deeds realize whatever balance there is, or isn't, between your body's strength and your heart's love. Between your heart chakra and your third eye is the center in your throat, the center of your words, your communication. Your words realize the balance, or the lack of it, between your heart's love and your mind's clarity.

Your deeds and your words are the 10,000 that are born out of the Three. And all 10,000 are still out in front of you. All the deeds and words that you are still ashamed of for the absence of balance they betray. And all the words and deeds you are still proud of for the love and balance they display. All 10,000 are still out in front of you. A wall. Let all 10,000 settle and empty into the Tao as you breathe out. And let those three centers you face the world with empty into the Tao. And the two deep inside Heart and Mind. And the One. Let everything settle and empty back into the Tao.

The Circles

Now that you have worked on your own pathways and centers and their connections we are going to get in circles in which we will connect these centers with others.

Sit close to the left of one of the participants, your left heel under your perineum and your right foot in front of your left. Your left knee is flat on the floor and your right knee is raised. Have the participant sit the same way, his left knee under your raised right knee, your right thigh across his Hara. Have everyone sit this way as close as possible in circles of eight to ten people, male and female alternating if possible. Have them slip rolled up towels or small cushions under their left buttocks.

Everybody sit close enough together to have your right knee overlapping the left knee of the person to your right. If possible sit on your own foot, your left heel pressing into your first chakra (in the perineum). Your right foot is on the floor in front of you, your bent right knee close to the hara of the person to your right. Move in even closer if possible. Cross your arms and reach out to the other side of the circle, each hand holding a different person's wrist. Lean back. Let the circle move you. Enjoy. Close your eyes. Continue letting the circle move you. Sit still.

Raise both your hands up in the air. Lower your left hand and hook the fingers of your left hand around the tailbone of the person to your left. Lower your right hand and place it over the sacrum of the person to your right. Straighten your back and feel the energy rising up your back.

Take a deep breath together...and let it all the way out. The next time you breathe in slowly slide your hand up the person to your right's spine. Stop when it reaches to just behind the Heart center. Hold it there and then, as you both breathe out, slide it back down to the sacrum. Continue sliding it up with each inbreath and down with each outbreath. Keep your left hand firmly hooked under the tailbone. Feel the rising up your own back as you breathe in and the opening in your heart all the way back down to the first chakra as you breathe out.

On the next inbreath slide your right hand all the way up to behind the throat and hold. Let whatever you feel rising up your back continue on out your throat as a sound, any sound. Slide your right hand back down to the sacrum. Rise up again on the next inbreath. Continue.

On the next inbreath slide your hand to just over the crown chakra. Without making any sound let what was rising up your spine rise higher and higher.

Keep your right hand over the crown and your left still hooked under the tailbone and lean forward into the circle. Feel how all your crowns join in the center.

Lift both your hands up. Place them on the far shoulders of those to each side of you. If you are the taller, your arms should cross over your neighbours'. Feel someone elses arms crossed with your arms behind your neighbours. Let go of the shoulders and hold the elbows of those other arms. You have linked arms with those who are sitting just beyond the people next to you.

Keep them firmly linked and sit up straight. Let your weight fall back and be supported by the circle of arms. Feel how you can completely let go and surrender into that circle. If the circle starts to move let it move you. Don't try to make it move. Surrender yourself to the circle.

Lower your hold on the arms to a place midway between the elbow and the wrist. Feel how the circle has grown. Enjoy whatever movement carries you.

If everyone is leaning back, surrendering their weight into the circle, it should start moving spontaneously, joyfully. If it doesn't, encourage them to let go more.

Lower your hold on the arms to the wrists.

Here the movement can get really wild. When the circle seems to be on the point of collapse say

Let go of the hands and fall back onto the floor.

Raise up both knees keeping them bent and your feet on the floor. Scoot towards the center until your knees are wedged between the knees of those to each side of you. Stretch your arms along the floor up over your head. Rest a moment.

Raise and bend your legs letting your knees drop towards your chest. Keeping your arms straight and close together swing them up and drop them between your knees. Cross your arms reaching under the backs of your knees. Hold the wrist of your neighbors hand that you find there. Keeping hold of the circle with your hands, let your arms and legs completely relax. Feel how open your first chakra is...and connected to the circle. Let go the hands. Keeping your knees bent, lower your feet back onto the floor.

Raise both your hands into the air. Place your left hand on the Hara (just below the navel) of the person to your left and your right hand on the Heart chakra of the person to your right, your arms relaxed and in comfortable positions.

Feel the rise and fall of the centers under your hands. It is the rise and fall of waves on an ocean. An ocean that it feels wonderful to be floating and drifting on.

We have two chakras connected and now we are going to connect a third into the circle. Raise your right leg up into the air. Bend and slowly lower your right leg down the inside of the left leg of the person to your right letting the outside of your foot rest against their first chakra. Relax both your legs letting them lie open. Feel how your first chakras are connected into the circle. Breathe in together feeling the rising all the way up your back. Continue, feeling the connection of all your chakras...and the rising...

Give everyone plenty of time to experience this rising.

The next time you breathe in slowly lift your hand off the heart chakra and place it over the crown of the person to your right. Feel the rising all the way up your back. Feel the completeness of the circle.

Raise both your hands up into the air. They are holding a circle of light over the circle. Raise both your feet up. They are standing on that circle of light.

Place your hands on the floor beside you. Without opening your eyes sit up and scoot back just far enough so that there is no physical contact. Sit in a position which helps keep your back straight. Your eyes still closed, feel how you are still connected to the circle in each one of your chakras. And how they are all connected. As you breathe in feel the rising up your back. And how it keeps rising up to join the others over the center of the circle as at the top of a dome. A dome of light.

We are one at the center of that dome. A light shining out to all sides. Let that light pour back into you...back into the Tao as you breathe out. Let everything empty into the Tao...And rise up your back as you breathe in... The Tao gives birth to the One...and the One to the Two... All that we have been doing to connect and open the flows and centers of our energy here has been Tantra. There are many ways to practice Tantra. One particularly powerful way to practice it is with a lover...to join the Two into One...Imagine you are with a lover who is sitting on your lap, or whose lap you are sitting on. The Yin and the Yang are in all of us... the settling down the front and the rising up the back is a complete cycle in each one. But where it can be most easily accessed may differ. Those who are more yang may find it beginning in their first chakra and rising up their back. Those who are more yin may first feel the opening of their heart chakra, an opening that continues all the way down the front. Hold your lover close to your heart and enter that cycle of opening and rising wherever it is most easily accessible. As your chakras connect, your lover's opening draws your rising up even more powerfully...and your lover's rising opens and fills your heart. The cycle becomes more complete the more you connect. Feel this sense of completion now with your lover...and hold them a moment, their head resting on your heart center. Slowly part and, without touching, look into each other's eyes. You are still connected. Close your eyes. Let it all settle back into the Tao.

Tantra Of The Loving Hug

There are many ways to practice Tantra. As we have seen in the circle today, being able to connect our chakras is not limited to those we are intimate with. We can feel this kind of connection with anyone when we practice bodywork. We can also feel it when we hug someone. This is Tantra of the Loving Hug. We are going to practice it now. Keep your eyes closed and stand up. Get used to being on your feet again. Enjoy standing. With your eyes closed be aware of the whole circle. You are still connected to that circle. Breathe out letting everything settle into the Tao. Open your eyes. Come together, two lines facing each other. After we complete each hug this line will not move and this line will move one person to the right. The person at the right end of it will walk back to its beginning. (*if there are an odd number of participants designate the longer line as the one to move and add* When that person walks back he should wait one turn focusing on his connection to the group as a whole.) We will now start. Place your right hand on each others heart chakra and look into each others eyes. Take a deep breath and, as you breathe out, embrace, your knees touching, your left hand holding the base of your partner's spine and your right hand holding the back of their heart center. As your chakras connect and open feel the rising up your back. *Give them time to feel this and then say*: Step back and, without touching each other, look into each others eyes. You are still connected. Take a deep breath and, as you breathe out, close your eyes letting everything settle back into the Tao. As you breathe in open your eyes. This line now moves one person to the right.

Repeat the above instructions. Continue until everybody has hugged everybody in the line opposite. Then have each line divide into two facing lines, one moving, one not moving. Repeat and continue dividing the lines until everybody has hugged everybody. Bring them into one big hug in the center. Introduce a sound to which the others can add their own expressing the internal resonance of the whole circle. Have everybody sit down and share their experiences. When the sharing is complete, say,

Before we separate take a moment to close your eyes and review inside yourselves all you have felt in this circle....Now let everything settle and empty back into the Tao. Feel how wonderful it is to have a place that everything can empty into, a place we carry around wherever we go, where we can ground ourselves in the Tao. Feel again the rising up your back, the One being born out of the Tao,...And the Two out of the One...And the Three out of the Two...and the Ten Thousand.... Feel again how complete this cycle is in you...And the more complete you feel it in yourself the more you can experience and celebrate your connection to others...And the more you experience and celebrate your connection to others, the more complete you will feel in yourselves these movements and cycles and transformations of energy through which creation itself, is continuously recreated in each and every one of us...

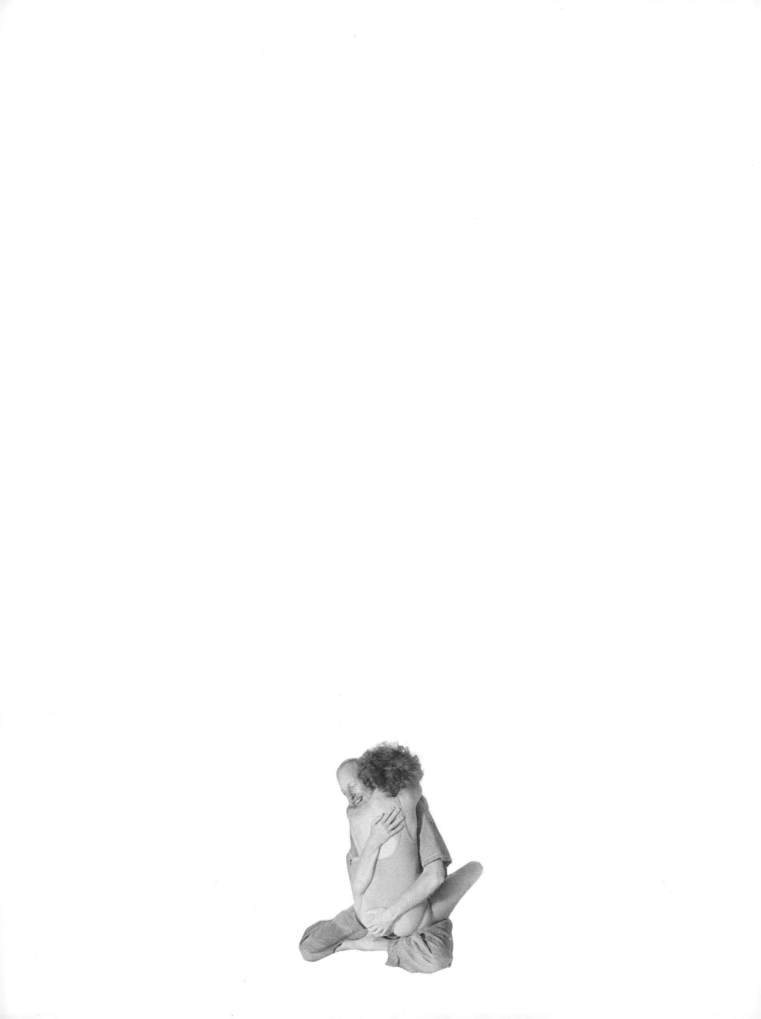